Classic Papers in Urology III

Classic Papers in Urology III

Edited by

Elmar W Gerharz
Staff Urologist, Department of Urology, Julius Maximilians-University Medical School, Würzburg, Germany

Mark Emberton
Senior Lecturer in Oncological Urology, Institute of Urology and Nephrology, University College, London, UK

Tim O'Brien
Consultant Urologist, Guy's and St Thomas' Hospitals, London, UK

Wyeth

Provided as a service to medicine by Wyeth

I S I S
MEDICAL
MEDIA

© 1999 by Isis Medical Media Ltd.
59 St. Aldates
Oxford OX1 1ST, UK

First published 1999
Reprinted in three parts 2000

British Library Cataloguing in Publication Data.
A catalogue record for this title is available from
the British Library

ISBN 1 899066 27 6

Gerharz, E. W. (Elmar)
Classic Papers in Urology
Elmar W Gerharz, Mark Emberton, Tim O'Brien (eds)

Always refer to the manufacturer's Prescribing
Information before prescribing drugs cited in this book.

Additional technical writing and editorial
services provided by Robert Reford (Oxford)

Typeset by
J&L Composition Ltd., Filey, North Yorkshire, UK

Image reproduction
Track Direct, London, UK

Isis Medical Media staff
Commissioning Editor: John Harrison
Editorial Controller: Fiona Cornell
Production Assistant: Sarah Sodhi

Printed and bound by
Giunti Industrie Grafiche, Italy

Distributed in the USA by
Books International Inc., P. O. Box 605,
Herndon, VA 20172, USA

Distributed in the rest of the world by
Plymbridge Distributors Ltd., Estover Road,
Plymouth PL6 7PY, UK

Contents

Part III

Contributors

Peter C. Albertsen
Associate Professor and Chief of Urology, Department of Surgery, University of Connecticut Health Center, Farmington, Connecticut, USA

Steven B. Brandes
Assistant Professor of Urologic Surgery, Washington University School of Medicine, St Louis, USA and Chief of Urology, St Louis VA Medical Center, St Louis, USA

Christopher S. Cooper
Assistant Professor, Pediatric Urology, Department of Urology, Children's Hospital of Iowa, Iowa City, Iowa, USA

Sakti Das
Professor of Urology, University of California Davis School of Medicine, California, USA

John P. Donohue
Distinguished Professor Emeritus of Urology, Indiana University, Indianapolis, Indiana, USA

Ahmed I. El-Sakka
Lecturer, Department of Urology, Ismailia, Egypt and Senior Registrar of Urology, Suez Canal University Hospital, Ismailia, Egypt

John M. Fitzpatrick
Professor of Surgery and Consultant Urologist, Chairman, Department of Surgery, Mater Misericordiae Hospital and University College, Dublin, Ireland

Norma Gibbons
Lecturer in Urology, University College Dublin and Mater Misericordiae Hospital, Dublin, Ireland

Marcus Hohenfellner
Associate Professor, Department of Urology, Johannes Gutenberg-University Medical School, Mainz, Germany

Rudolf Hohenfellner
Emeritus Professor of Urology, Department of Urology, Johannes Gutenberg-University Medical School, Mainz, Germany

Tom F. Lue
Professor, Department of Urology, University of California, San Francisco, USA and Chief of Urology, UCSF/Mt Zion Medical Center, California, USA

Jack W. McAninch
Professor, Department of Urology, University of California, Chief of Urology, San Francisco General Hospital, San Francisco, USA and Vice-Chairman, Department of Urology, University of California, San Francisco, USA

Anthony R. Mundy
Professor of Urology, Director of the Institute of Urology and Nephrology, London, UK

David J. Ralph
Consultant Urologist at St Peter's Hospital, London, UK and Honorary Senior Lecturer at Institute of Urology, University College, London, UK

Mark S. Soloway
Professor and Chairman, Department of Urology, University of Miami School of Medicine, Miami, Florida, USA

Howard M. Snyder, III
Professor, Division of Pediatric Urology, Children's Hospital of Philadelphia, Pennsylvania, USA

Joachim W. Thüroff
Professor and Chairman, Department of Urology, Johannes Gutenberg-University Medical School, Mainz, Germany

Justin Vale
Consultant Urologist, Department of Urology, St Mary's Hospital, London, UK and Honorary Clinical Senior Lecturer, Imperial College School of Medicine, London, UK

R. Dixon Walker
Professor and Chief of Urology, University of Florida College of Medicine, Gainesville, Florida, USA

Christopher R. J. Woodhouse
Reader in Adolescent Urology, The Institute of Urology and Nephrology, University College, London, UK

Hugh N. Whitfield
Reader in Urology, Institute of Urology and Nephrology, London, UK; Consultant Urologist, Central Middlesex Hospital, London, UK; Honorary Consultant Urologist, St Peter's Hospitals; Civilian Consultant to the Army in Urology; President, European Board of Urology

Foreword

Webster's Dictionary defines knowledge as 'understanding acquired through experience – the total or range of what has been perceived or learned'. Indeed, clinical urologists and urological researchers alike must first master existing knowledge, an educational process which occupies the first one-third of their life span. Only then can they hope to effectively manage patients or initiate research directed toward pushing forward the continually advancing frontiers of urological science upon which clinical care is based. Not unlike the coral reefs of our planet's tropical seas, current generations build upon the work of their forebears.

This publication is timely and unique. It constitutes the first effort to chronicle in a single compendium those works upon which contemporary urological science and its therapies are based. It is not retrospective historical prose written by a person or persons whose interpretations of the past are coloured by bias and personal opinions. It is, in point of fact, a superb history of the science of our profession based upon the original work of distinguished authors. The only subjective aspect was the selection of papers within each of the fifteen areas of urology deserving the distinction of being deemed 'classic'. Yet even here, it is an open process. The reviewers have expressed their reasons for inclusion and their personal views as to the strengths and weaknesses of the selected works, thus making the reader privy to the selection process.

As the editors state in their introduction, the reader of this volume may disagree with which manuscripts were selected as classics. One or more of the reader's personal historic 'greats' may have been excluded. Nonetheless, I find it difficult to argue with the included selections. For within these pages resides a review of literature upon which much, if not all, our current urological measurement is based.

The editors and the publisher are to be commended for conceiving this significant undertaking. The reviewers are to be complimented upon the end product of their enormous task of literature review – a task taking them back over decades of time and volumes of literature. If it is true that the past is prologue – and I truly believe it is – this edition should be required reading for all of us who strive to provide urological services to society and for those who labour in the research arena. For as we undertake our professional responsibilities, we stand upon the shoulders of the giants who proceeded us – much of whose pivotal work is included herein.

Finally, I should like to thank Mr Mark Emberton, the editors and the publishers for the honour of allowing me to contribute these comments as a foreword to what is clearly a classic in its own right.

H. Logan Holtgrewe, MD
Associate Professor of Urology
Johns Hopkins University, Baltimore, MD, USA;
Former President, American Urological Association;
Past President, The American Board of Urology

Foreword

With the advent of modern information and communication technology we are currently witnessing not only the agony of the good old-fashioned textbook but also a process that generates an information load of mind blowing dimension. In these exciting times, in which the physician loses his status of being a 'knower' to become a 'navigator' instead, it is more important than ever to point out the buoys and the landmarks, the stars and the lighthouses.

This book is about orientation, or to put it better, it is about leading the way. Spanning almost 150 years of innovative power in urology this compelling anthology has it all: the legendary names, Huggins and Hodges, Turner-Warwick, Burch and Einhorn, Mitrofanoff and Kock, and the ingenious concepts, ESWL, BCG, ICSI and PSA.

In an unusual presentation – not drowned in endless textbook chapters – the classic papers come with thoughtful, occasionally philosophical comments by an exquisite panel of experts, some of whom are legends in their own right. Who else but John Donohue could have selected the papers on testicular cancer, who could compete with Jack McAninch, the 'inventor' of urological trauma?

A unique mixture of familiar and new, classic and innovative, names and ideas, philosophy and humour may even render this book a 'cult' text changing the routine of urological board exams.

I regard it as a distinct privilege to add the above thoughts as a foreword to *Classic Papers in Urology* and hope that this opus will reach the target population it deserves: all those dedicated to the care of patients, research and teaching in urology. Textbooks go out of date and fashion, classic papers never will.

Hubertus Riedmiller, MD
Professor of Urology, Head and Chairman,
Julius Maximilians-University Medical School, Würzburg, Germany

Introduction

No serious study of literature would be possible without some reference to the great works. An expert without first hand knowledge of Shakespeare, Milton, Tolstoy, Melville and many, many more would struggle to put modern work into any sort of historical context. Yet in any particular medical discipline there exists a similar body of work that is generally acknowledged to be the key piece of work in that area. Although these works are often quoted and their first (or possibly last) authors are revered, they are seldom read. We tend instead to read the new, the exciting, the controversial – not the familiar. Computers and electronic literature searches have made things worse. A trip to the library now, more often than not, involves a session in front of a screen which might well be in a bedroom, an on-line cafe, or a remote corner of a hospital. Because of this it takes a huge amount of effort to go to a library and pull out dusty volumes that pre-date inclusion onto the on-line search engines. For more recent papers the abstract on screen is so much more accessible than a paper which is not held in a local library – so we tend to use it instead.

The privileged few who are able to enjoy complete articles tend to fall into two groups. The first is the researcher who is trying to become an expert in a particular field and identifies and retrieves all the papers in one particular area. The second is the clinician who gets together with like minded colleagues to form a Journal Club. It was during one of these Journal Clubs at the Institute of Urology in London that the idea for this book was generated. Were there any books available that identified and appraised the great papers in Urology? asked one of the students. "No", we said. But the idea was born.

There is no right way to identify a 'Classic Paper'. No two experts will agree on all of them. And a year from now today's 'Classic Paper' might need demoting, whilst others will be pushing for the title 'Classic'. In this book we have invited experts to confer the title 'Classic' to a particular paper. Each expert was asked to identify what they considered to be the top ten papers in their own specialist area. Once identified the experts were required to state why they considered the paper a 'Classic' and also highlight any methodological problems with the paper according to a pre-defined template. Although this approach lies at the heart of this book we have also generated league tables of the most cited papers – both in raw form and adjusted for date of publication. A recent paper will not have had the equivalent time in the public domain for it to become a commonly cited paper than a paper published several years earlier. We were keen to see whether there existed any correlation between the papers cited by our team of experts and their rank in the league table of published work. We, and for this we will have to wait, were also keen to see how the citation rankings as well as the 'Classic Papers' will change with time.

To help the reader use this book we have asked our expert selectors to tell us how they went about picking ten papers out of the almost infinite number available (30 000 papers on prostate cancer since 1966). Each selector describes what criteria were used. Some choose from each broad discipline: epidemiology, prevention, clinical diagnosis, operative technique, clinical trials and basic science. Some highlighted papers that defined new diseases or treatments, others described papers that changed our whole way of thinking about a disease, a few felt that only those papers that have stood the test of time were worthy of inclusion. All said they enjoyed the exercise and found it singularly illuminating going back over the building bricks of our knowledge base.

We hope that these 'Classic Papers' will stimulate an enjoyable debate. No doubt many of you will disagree with our experts and we would hope that you will formulate your own. Perhaps some of you will be encouraged to seek out some of the original texts to read as we did ourselves. Some of you will perhaps be sufficiently inspired by some of these papers and will set about writing a 'Classic Paper' for inclusion in the next issue.

Elmar Gerharz, Mark Emberton and Timothy O' Brien

CHAPTER 12

Erectile dysfunction

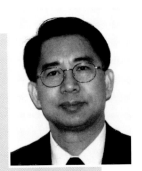

TOM F LUE, MD, FACS

- 1965–1972: Medical School, Kaohsiung Medical College, Taiwan
- 1978–1981: Urology residency, SUNY Downstate Medical Center, Brooklyn, New York, USA
- 1992–present: Professor of Urology, University of California, San Francisco, USA
- 1996–present: Chief of Urology, UCSF/Mt Zion Medical Center, California, USA

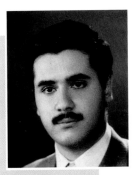

AHMED I EL-SAKKA, MD

- 1981–1988: Medical School: Suez Canal University, Ismailia, Egypt
- 1991–1994: Resident of Urology, Suez Canal University Hospital, Ismailia, Egypt
- 1998–present: Lecturer of Urology, Suez Canal University, Ismailia, Egypt
- 1998–present: Senior Registrar of Urology, Suez Canal University Hospital, Ismailia, Egypt

Introduction

We have selected the pioneering and most influential papers on different aspects of impotence research. The first shows convincing evidence of venous compression (not constriction) as an essential component of penile erection. The second establishes nitric oxide as the predominant neurotransmitter for penile erection. The third helps us to understand how the millions of smooth muscle cells in the penis can work together during erection. These three papers changed our concept and led to exploration of molecular pathways of erection. The next two brought us more accurate methods for assessing penile arterial and venous function, and the sixth introduces nocturnal penile erection monitoring as a classic test to rule out psychogenic impotence. The seventh/eighth introduces the concept of revascularization of the penis. The ninth presents evidence that intracavernous injection therapy can be used to treat impotence. The tenth shows that a transurethral approach can also be effective. The final paper is the first report showing that sildenafil can be used to treat organic or mixed impotence with excellent results and thus ushers in a new era in impotence treatment.

Title

Mechanisms of venous occlusion during canine penile erection: an anatomic demonstration

Authors

Fournier GR Jr, Juenemann KP, Lue TF, Tanagho EA

Reference

Journal of Urology 1987; **137**: 163–167

Abstract

Hemodynamic studies have clearly demonstrated that intracorporeal injection of papaverine causes an increase of venous outflow resistance, and we therefore undertook a study of the venous drainage of the canine penis to delineate the anatomic changes in the venular structure during papaverine-induced erection.

In 11 dogs, the corpora were examined by corrosion casting in six and serial trichrome staining and histologic sectioning in five. Low-power scanning electron microscopy of the corrosion casts demonstrated the existence of a venular plexus interposed between the tunica albuginea and the sinusoidal spaces. After papaverine injection, this subalbugineal venular plexus is compressed between the dilated sinusoids from below and the tunic albuginea from above, such that venous drainage is effectively impeded. Examination of two cadaveric human penile corrosion casts by low-power scanning electron microscopy revealed evidence of a similar subalbugineal venular plexus draining in to the emissary veins along the shaft of the penis.

Based on the above, a model for the anatomic basis of venous occlusion during penile erection is outlined. Along with arteriolar and sinusoidal smooth-muscle relaxation, this can account for the three basic hemodynamic changes necessary for erection: increased arterial inflow, increased intracorporeal pressure, and increased venous outflow resistance.

Summary

This study was designed to demonstrate the mechanism of venous drainage of the canine penis and to delineate the anatomical changes in the structure of the veins during papaverine-induced erection. The corpora cavernosa were examined in six dogs by corrosion casting, and by trichrome staining and histological sectioning in five. Scanning electron microscopy of the corrosion casts demonstrated the existence of a venular plexus interposed between the tunica albuginea and the sinusoidal spaces. After papaverine injection, this subalbugineal venular plexus is compressed between the dilated sinusoids from below and the tunica albuginea from above. Examination of two penile corrosion casts from human cadavers revealed evidence of a similar subalbugineal venular plexus.

Citation count	128

Related reference (1)	Ebbehoj J, Wagner G. Insufficient penile erection due to abnormal drainage of cavernous bodies. *Urology* 1979; **13**: 507–510.

Related reference (2)	Shirai M, Ishii N, Mitsukawa S, Matsuda S, Nakamura M. Hemodynamic mechanism of erection in the human penis. *Archives of Andrology* 1978; **1**: 345–349.

Related reference (3)	Banya Y, Ushiki T, Takagane H, Aoki H, Kubo T, Ohhori T, Ide C. Two circulatory routes within the human corpus cavernosum penis: a scanning electron microscopic study of corrosion casts. *Journal of Urology* 1989; **142**: 879–883.

Key message

Veno-occlusion during penile erection is a result of compression of subtunical venules between the distended sinusoids and the tunica albuginea. It is not due to vasoconstriction as suggested in the past.

Why it's important

This is the first detailed experimental study to demonstrate the mechanism of venous occlusion during erection. This report also described the changes in the venular architecture of the canine penis, subsequent to papaverine-induced penile erection. A model is then proposed that integrates the haemodynamic events with the penile anatomical structures.

Strengths

1. Strong methodology showing the mechanism of venous occlusion.
2. This report helps towards better understanding of the mechanism of penile erection.
3. Clear and readable format.

Weakness

1. The methodology was different in human casting; however, this may result partly from free intercommunication between the two corporeal bodies in the human. Moreover, work on cadavers with stagnant circulation is different from the running circulation in live dogs.

Relevance

This study demonstrates for the first time how the venous system works in coordination with arterial and sinusoidal smooth muscle to produce an erection.

Title

Nitric oxide and cyclic GMP formation upon electrical field stimulation cause relaxation of corpus cavernosum smooth muscle

Authors

Ignarro LJ, Bush PA, Buga GM, Wood KS, Fukuto JM, Rajfer J

Reference

Biochemical and Biophysical Research Communications 1990; **170**: 843–850

Abstract

In the presence of functional adrenergic and cholinergic blockade, electrical field stimulation relaxes corpus cavernosum smooth muscle by unknown mechanisms. We report here that electrical field stimulation of isolated strips of rabbit corpus cavernosum promotes the endogenous formation and release of nitric oxide (NO), nitrite, and cyclic GMP. Corporal smooth muscle relaxation in response to electrical field stimulation, in the presence of guanethidine and atropine, was abolished by tetrodotoxin and potassium-induced depolarization, and was markedly inhibited by N^G-nitro-L-arginine, N^G-amino-L-arginine, oxyhemoglobin, and methylene blue, but was unaffected by indomethacin. The inhibitory effects of N^G-substituted analogs of L-arginine were nearly completely reversed by addition of excess L-arginine but not D-arginine. Corporal smooth muscle relaxation elicited by electrical field stimulation was accompanied by rapid and marked increases in tissue levels of nitrite and cyclic GMP, and all responses were nearly abolished by N^G-nitro-L-arginine. These observations indicate that penile erection may be mediated by NO generated in response to nonadrenergic-noncholinergic neurotransmission.

Summary

The authors reported that electrical field stimulation (EFS) of isolated strips of rabbit corpus cavernosum promotes the endogenous formation and release of nitric oxide (NO), nitrite and cyclic GMP. They concluded that penile erection may be mediated by NO generated in response to nonadrenergic, non-cholinergic (NANC) neurotransmission.

Citation count	237

Related reference (1)

Rajfer J, Aronson WJ, Bush PA, Dorey FJ, Ignarro LJ. Nitric oxide as a mediator of relaxation of the corpus cavernosum in response to nonadrenergic, noncholinergic neurotransmission. *New England Journal of Medicine* 1992; **326**: 90–94.

Related reference (2)

Kim N, Azadzoi KM, Goldstein I, Saenz de Tejada I. A nitric oxide-like factor mediates nonadrenergic-noncholinergic neurogenic relaxation of penile corpus cavernosum smooth muscle. *Journal of Clinical Investigation* 1991; **88**: 112–118.

Related reference (3)   Burnett AL, Lowenstein CJ, Bredt DS, Chang TS, Snyder SH. Nitric oxide: a physiologic mediator of penile erection. *Science* 1992; **257**: 401–403.

Key message

Penile erection may be mediated by nitric oxide generated in response to non-adrenic, non-cholinergic transmission.

Why it's important

This is a thorough study demonstrating the mechanism by which EFS causes relaxation of the corpus cavernosum. The experimental evidence supports the hypothesis that relaxation elicited by EFS is the result of NANC neuron-dependent formation of NO. Moreover, the inhibitors of NO markedly inhibited EFS-induced relaxation. This and several other studies helped to establish the role of NO as a principal neurotransmitter in penile erection.

Strengths

1. A controlled methodology for studying the NANC mechanism of erection.
2. Informative results that opened the door for further basic and clinical studies.

Weaknesses

1. There is no correlation between the in vitro and the in vivo functional studies.
2. Further functional study of in vivo NO or the NO producer may help further the understanding of the mechanism of NO action.

Relevance

This is an exemplary study and the results were reproduced extensively by others.

Title

Gap junctions formed of connexin 43 are found between smooth muscle cells of human corpus cavernosum

Authors

Campos De Carvalho AC, Roy C, Moreno AP, Melma A, Hertzberg EL, Christ GJ, Spray DC

Reference

Journal of Urology 1993; **149**: 1568–1575

Abstract

Despite sparse autonomic innervation, the smooth muscle cells of the corpus cavernosum relax and contract synchronously to achieve penile erection and flaccidity. As with other smooth muscle cell types, the excitation process in the corpora is presumably propagated through gap junctions to allow the diffusions of current-carrying ions and second messenger molecules from cell to cell. Using both molecular and immunocytochemical techniques, we have identified gap junctions between human corporal smooth muscle cells in situ and in culture. Northern analyses demonstrated that corporal smooth muscle cells express the gap junction protein connexin43 isoforms, but not connexin26 mRNA. Immunoblots showed the presence of connexin43 isoforms, whereas connexin32 was not detected. Immunocytochemical studies in cultured cells identified prominent connexin43 immunoreactive puncta between cells, as well as within the cytoplasm. In addition, gap junction membranes both in situ and in culture were labelled in thin section by anti-connexin43 antibodies using the immunogold technique. We conclude that the presence and distribution of gap junctions in this sparsely innervated tissue may provide an important mechanism of intercellular communication among the smooth muscle cells, and thus play a major role in coordinating tissue contraction and relaxation.

Summary

Using both molecular and immunocytochemical techniques, authors have identified gap junctions between human corporeal smooth muscle cells both *in situ* and in culture. Corporeal smooth muscle cells expressed the mRNA of gap junction protein connexin 43, but not of connexin 26 mRNA. Immunoblots showed the presence of connexin 43 isoforms, whereas connexin 32 was not detected. Immunocytochemical study in cultured cells confirmed the results.

Citation count	32
Related reference (1)	Brink PR. Gap junctions in vascular smooth muscle. *Acta Physiologica Scandinavia* 1998; **164**: 349–356.
Related reference (2)	Moreno AP, Campos de Carvalho AC, Christ G, Melman A, Spray DC. Gap junctions between human corpus cavernosum smooth muscle cells: gating properties and unitary conductance. *American Journal of Physiology* 1993; **264**: C80–92.
Related reference (3)	Christ GJ, Moreno AP, Melman A, Spray DC. Gap junction-mediated intercellular diffusion of Ca^{2+} in cultured human corporal smooth muscle cells. *American Journal of Physiology* 1992; **263**: C373–383.

Key message

This paper helps towards better understanding of the mechanisms of intercellular communication among the cavernosal smooth muscle cells, and the mechanisms of coordination and synergism in contraction and relaxation processes.

Why it's important

This is the first report identifying the gap junctions between corporeal smooth muscle cells *in situ* and in culture, and the first to localize connexin 43 to these junctional regions at the electron microscopic level. This study supports the hypothesis that the excitation process in the corpora is propagated through gap junctions, to allow the spread of electric current and second messenger molecules from cell to cell.

Strengths

1. An interesting idea studied with a good methodology.
2. Clear and readable format.
3. Informative results.

Weakness

1. The paper did not discuss the relevance of the findings for clinical application adequately.

Relevance

The gap junctions in the corporeal smooth muscle may be a potential target to enhance smooth muscle relaxation and to promote erection.

Title

Vasculogenic impotence evaluated by high-resolution ultrasonography and pulsed Doppler spectrum analysis

Authors

Lue TF, Hricak H, Larich KW, Tanagho EA

Reference

Radiology 1985; **155**: 777–781

Abstract

Vasculogenic impotence was evaluated by high-resolution sonography and quantitative Doppler spectrum analysis in 21 patients and two normal volunteers. Erection was induced by intracorporeal injection of papaverine, and B-scan imaging and Doppler analysis were performed with the penis flaccid and erect. The corpora cavernosa and its deep arteries, median septum, and corpus spongiosum were clearly displayed in every subject, with the dorsal vein and dorsal artery seen ventral to the corpora cavernosa. In the flaccid state, in all subjects, Doppler analysis demonstrated flow in the dorsal arteries but not in the deep arteries. During erection, the B-mode image showed varying degrees of enlargement of the corpora cavernosa, with increased tissue echogenicity, as well as hypoechoic area in the peri-arterial region. The diameter of the penile arteries and flow within them also increased by varying degrees. Quantification of blood flow through all deep and dorsal arteries is feasible with this technique.

Summary

Vasculogenic impotence was evaluated by high-resolution sonography and quantitative Doppler spectrum analysis in 21 patients and two normal volunteers. Doppler analysis was performed with the penis both flaccid and erect. Doppler analysis showed flow in the dorsal arteries but not in the deep arteries in the flaccid state. During erection, the diameter of the penile arteries and flow within them increased by varying degrees.

Citation count	179

Related reference (1)	Michal V, Pospíchal J. Phalloarteriography in the diagnosis of erectile impotence. *World Journal of Surgery* 1978; **2**: 239–248.
Related reference (2)	Schwartz AN, Wang KY, Mack LA, Lowe M, Berger RE, Cyr DR, Feldman M. Evaluation of normal erectile function with color flow Doppler sonography. *American Journal of Roentgenology* 1989; **153**: 1155–1160.
Related reference (3)	Martins FE, Padma-Nathan H. Diffuse veno-occlusive dysfunction: the underlying hemodynamic abnormality resulting in failure to respond to intracavernous pharmacotherapy. *Journal of Urology* 1996; **156**: 1942–1946.

Key message

This is the first description of a non-invasive technique that can accurately assess the anatomical and functional aspects of penile arteries.

Why it's important

This technique is a significant addition to the armamentarium for the diagnosis of arterial impotence. Before the development of this non-invasive, less complicated and safe technique, arteriography, which is invasive and not without complications, was the only diagnostic tool.

Strengths

1. An example of a good idea that is easy to learn and perform.
2. The technique is now accepted as a standard diagnostic method in impotence practices.

Weaknesses

1. The number of subjects is too small to make a normative value for this new technique.
2. The technique is somewhat more complicated than the current procedure; however, this may result in part from the early experiences of this new test and the stage of the duplex Doppler machine's technology.

Relevance

The introduction of a duplex Doppler technique to impotence practice allowed better diagnosis of arteriogenic impotence, without the need to perform arteriography.

Title

In vivo assessment of trabecular smooth muscle tone, its application in pharmaco-cavernosometry and analysis of intracavernous pressure determinants

Authors

Hatzichristou DG, Saenz De Tejada I, Kupferman A, Namburi S, Pescatori ES, Udelson D, Goldstein I

Reference

Journal of Urology 1995; **153**: 1126–1135

Abstract

A pharmaco-cavernosometry based clinical study was designed to define hemodynamic parameters consistent with complete trabecular smooth muscle relaxation, establish a methodology for overcoming incomplete trabecular smooth muscle relaxation, and determine under controlled conditions the contribution of venous outflow and arterial inflow to the steady-state equilibrium intracavernous pressure. Flow-pressure relationships were analyzed in 21 patients, each of whom was assumed to have complete smooth muscle relaxation by virtue of the full, rigid and maintained erectile response following intracavernous vasodilator administration, which required intracavernous adrenergic agonists to achieve detumescence. Flow-to-maintain values increased linearly with intracavernous pressure while venous outflow resistance values were high and constant. Based on these relationships, trabecular smooth muscle tone was assessed in 123 impotent patients. In 14%, 63% and 14% of the patients (112 of 123 overall), respectively, 1, 2 and 3 doses of vasoactive agents were required to achieve hemodynamic relationships consistent with complete trabecular smooth muscle relaxation. In 9% of the patients such hemodynamic relationships were unable to be reached. In the 112 patients the influence of different engineering based measures of corporeal veno-occlusive function, including flow-to-maintain, pressure decay, venous outflow resistance and corporeal capacitance, was analyzed against the spectrum of equilibrium steady-stage intracavernous pressures. Two distinct equilibrium pressure groups were identified reflecting different capacitance states: pressures greater than 60 mm Hg (associated with low capacitance values) and pressures less than 50 mm Hg (associated with high capacitance values), with pressures 50 to 59 mm Hg representing a hemodynamic transition zone. When analyzed during complete trabecular smooth muscle relaxation, corporeal veno-occlusive hemodynamic variables in conjunction with cavernous arterial perfusion pressure determine the steady-state equilibrium intracavernous pressure. Failure to assess corporeal veno-occlusive function under such conditions will overestimate the degree of suspected corporeal structural disease.

Summary

This study was designed to define the haemodynamic parameters influencing complete trabecular smooth muscle relaxation and to establish a methodology for overcoming incomplete trabecular smooth muscle relaxation. Two distinct equilibrium pressure groups were identified, reflecting low and high capacitance states: (1) pressure greater than 60 mmHg associated with low capacitance values; and (2) pressure less than 50 mmHg associated with high capacitance values. The authors concluded that failure to assess the corporeal veno-occclusive function under complete trabecular smooth muscle relaxation will overestimate the degree of suspected disease of the corporeal structures.

Citation count   19

Related reference (1)   Virag R, Spencer PP, Frydman D. Artificial erection in diagnosis and treatment of impotence. *Urology* 1984; **24**: 157–161.

Related reference (2)   Wespes E, Delcour C, Struyven J, Schulman CC. Cavernometry–cavernography: its role in organic impotence. *European Urology* 1984; **10**: 229–232.

Related reference (3)   Lue, TF, Hricak H, Schmidt RA, Tanagho EA. Functional evaluation of penile veins by cavernosography in papaverine induced erection. *Journal of Urology* 1986; **135**: 479–482.

Key message

Complete trabecular smooth muscle relaxation is mandatory in the assessment of veno-occlusive function and can be obtained by repeated injections of vasoactive agents.

Why it's important

This study delineates the mandatory circumstances that should be attained before performing cavernosometry; therefore, diminution of the inherent pitfalls of this technique is possible and reproducible data can be obtained.

Strengths

1. Excellent methodology for studying the circumstances necessary for using cavernosometry.
2. This study provides a method for validation of a hitherto non-standardized technique.

Weakness

1. Use of many statistical analyses and engineering-based measurements is sometimes confusing and not easy to understand.

Relevance

The article provides a convincing argument and a useful technique to achieve complete smooth muscle relaxation during pharmaco-cavernosometry.

Title

A simple and inexpensive transducer for quantitative measurements of penile erection during sleep

Authors

Karakan I

Reference

Behavioural and Research Methods and Instrumentation 1969; **1**(7): 251–252

Abstract

Not available

Summary

The construction of a mercury strain-gauge transducer for measuring penile erection and scoring rules for tumescent episodes were described. The gauge device has been found to be inexpensive, reliable and easy to construct. It is capable of transducing changes in circumference in the penis of adults and infants, the clitoris of patients with congenital adrenal hyperplasia and the nipples of women.

Citation count	Not available
Related reference (1)	Karakan I. Nocturnal penile tumescence as a biologic marker in assessing erectile dysfunction. *Psychosomatics* 1982; **23**: 349–360.
Related reference (2)	Bradley WE, Timm GW, Gallagher JM, Johnson BK. New method for continuous measurement of nocturnal penile tumescence and rigidity. *Urology* 1985; **26**: 4–9.
Related reference (3)	Levine LA, Carroll RA. Nocturnal penile tumescence and rigidity in men without complaints of erectile dysfunction using a new quantitative analysis software. *Journal of Urology* 1994; **152**: 1103–1107.

Key message

This is the first reliable method for measuring nocturnal penile erection after many previous unsuccessful trials and methods.

Why it's important

The author's pioneering work in this field elucidates the mechanisms of erection during sleep. The simple method described in this report is the basis for more sophisticated equipment used for the same purpose. The idea of measuring nocturnal penile tumescence became a focus of interest for many researchers working in this field.

Strengths

1. An example of a good idea turned into a simple method for clinical application.
2. With more technological refinement, this test became a standard investigative tool for differentiation between organic and non-organic impotence in patients who are indistinguishable symptomatically.

Weaknesses

1. The author did not include the results that support the use of this transducer, but merely mentioned his conclusions.
2. No detailed description of the method of using this technique, or its limitations and potential pitfalls.

Relevance

This report provides a relevant method for measuring nocturnal penile tumescence and, with more refinement, this test became a useful clinical tool for diagnosis of impotence.

Title

Arterial epigastricocavernous anastomosis for the treatment of sexual impotence

Authors

Michal V, Kramár R, Pospíchal J, Hejhal L

Reference

World Journal of Surgery 1977; **1**: 515–519.

Abstract

Not available

Summary

This paper discusses the different methods of revascularization of corporeal bodies. The first technique addressed was epigastricocavernous anastomosis in 32 patients, and the results were not encouraging because only 10 patients could resume sexual activity. However, 3–11 months after the operation, all patent anastomoses became occluded. The second technique was femoropudendal bypass using a saphenous vein graft in two patients; however, the anastomosis was occluded in both of them in less than a year; these results limit the utility of this technique. Finally, they discussed the technique of epigastricopenile anastomosis (epigastric artery to dorsal penile artery) in 18 patients; the anastomosis remained patent in 10 patients for more than 6 months.

Citation count	89

Related reference (1)	Virag R, Saltiel H, Floresco J, Shoukry K, Dufour B. Surgical treatment of vascular impotence by arterialization of the dorsal vein of the penis. Experience of 292 cases. *Chirurgie* 1988; **114**: 703–714.
Related reference (2)	Goldstein I. Overview of types and results of vascular surgical procedures for impotence. *Cardiovascular and Interventional Radiology* 1988; **11**: 240–244.
Related reference (3)	Hauri D. Revascularization of the penis in cases of male impotence of vascular origin. *Annales d'Urologie* 1993; **27**: 144–151.

Key message

The authors concluded that, physiologically, the epigastricopenile anastomosis is superior to the other procedures and seems to hold better prospects for long-term potency.

Why it's important

This report addressed, in an objective manner, the different methods of penile revascularization, and demonstrated the drawbacks and pitfalls of each technique. It also provided insights into the new era of using microvascular techniques to revascularize the penis. The technique (epigastric artery to dorsal penile artery) subsequently became one of the standard techniques in penile revascularization.

Strengths

1. Informative report discussing, in a clear manner, different techniques to revascularize the penis.
2. Clear and readable format.

Weaknesses

1. The number of patients was not enough to derive a final conclusion about the validity of each technique.
2. The time of follow-up for the epigastricopenile anastomosis is short.
3. There are no definite indications or criteria for selection of patients for penile revascularization.

Relevance

This is a relevant report demonstrating the basic techniques of penile revascularization. In spite of the advances in the management of erectile dysfunction using more conservative methods, penile revascularization plays an important role in the management of impotence.

Title

Management of erectile impotence: use of implantable inflatable prosthesis

Authors

Brantley Scott F, Bradley WE, Timm GW

Reference

Urology 1973; **2**: 80–82

Abstract

Not available

Summary

An implantable, inflatable, penile prosthesis for the treatment of organic erectile dysfunction has been described in this report. The preliminary results were encouraging, in terms of success in achieving vaginal penetration.

Citation count	199

Related reference (1)	Small MP, Carrion HM, Gordon JA. Small–Carrion penile prosthesis. New implant for management of impotence. *Urology* 1975; **5**: 479–486.
Related reference (2)	Jonas U, Jacobi GH. Silicone–silver penile prosthesis: description, operative approach and results. *Journal of Urology* 1980; **123**: 865–867.
Related reference (3)	Timm GW. Mechanical penile prostheses. The OmniPhase and DuraPhase designs. *Asaio Transactions* 1988; **34**: 996–998.

Key message

Revolutionary changes are expected to take place in both design and construction of the device as well as in surgical technique, if long-term results are satisfactory.

Why it's important

This is the first report to describe the use of an inflatable penile prosthesis that offered an excellent solution in properly selected patients. A more natural appearance and mechanical erectile function can be achieved with this type of prosthesis. More importantly, pressure necrosis caused by the tight prosthesis can be avoided and the cosmetic concealment of the prosthesis can be assured.

Strengths

1. With more technological refinement, this kind of prosthesis has become the most preferable form for patients nowadays.
2. Clear and readable format.

Weaknesses

1. The number of patients included in this report was not sufficient to reach a final conclusion about the validity of this kind of penile prosthesis.
2. The time of follow-up at the time of writing this paper was too short to evaluate the patients' and partners' satisfaction.

Relevance

This kind of prosthesis attained a lot of interest from the patients and their partners, and became a more popular prosthesis than those described in the past.

Title

Intracavernous injection of papaverine for erectile failure

Author

Virag R

Reference

The Lancet 1982; **ii**: 938

Abstract

Not available

Summary

Accidental intracavernous injection of papaverine during a surgical shunting procedure produced a prolonged and fully rigid erection. The preliminary findings relate to 15 organic cases and 10 non-organic cases. The immediate reaction after intracorporeal injection of papaverine was a significant increase in intracorporeal pressure. Seven of the fifteen patients with an organic aetiology reported significantly improved erection in the days following the procedure, but none of the non-organic cases reported any changes in their erectile capability.

Citation count	341

Related reference (1)	Zorgniotti AW, Lefleur RS. Auto-injection of the corpus cavernosum with a vasoactive drug combination for vasculogenic impotence. *Journal of Urology* 1985; **133**: 39–41.
Related reference (2)	Ishii N, Watanabe H, Irisawa C, Kikuchi Y, Kawamura S, Suzuki K *et al.* [Studies on male sexual impotence. Report 18. Therapeutic trial with prostaglandin E1 for organic impotence] *Nippon Hinyokika Gakkai Zasshi* [*Japanese Journal of Urology*] 1986; **77**: 954–962.
Related reference (3)	Linet OI, Ogrinc FG. Efficacy and safety of intracavernosal alprostadil in men with erectile dysfunction. The Alprostadil Study Group. *New England Journal of Medicine* 1996; **334**: 873–877.

Key message

Intracorporeal injection of papaverine induces penile erection.

Why it's important

This method of inducing erection revolutionized the diagnosis and treatment of erectile dysfunction.

Strength

1. Although the results were preliminary, this report was convincing and showed a promising method of treatment for the future.

Weaknesses

1. The results were not based on a prospective, randomized, double-blind, placebo-controlled study.
2. The number of patients in this report was small.
3. There was no explanation for why none of the non-organic impotent patients experienced any improvement after papaverine injection.

Relevance

Although it is not a complete study and is just a report in the form of a letter to the editor, the results were relevant and this drug has since been used for intracorporeal injection.

Title

Treatment of men with erectile dysfunction with transurethral alprostadil. Medicated Urethral System for Erection (MUSE) Study Group

Authors

Padma-Nathan H, Hellstrom WJ, Kaiser FE, Labasky RF, Lue TF, Nolten WE, Norwood PC, Peterson CA, Shabsigh R, Tam PY

Reference

New England Journal of Medicine 1997; **336**: 1–7

Abstract

Background: erectile dysfunction in men is common. We evaluated a system by which alprostadil (prostaglandin E_1) is delivered transurethrally to treat this disorder.

Methods: alprostadil was delivered transurethrally in a double-blind, placebo-controlled study of 1511 men, 27 to 88 years of age, who had chronic erectile dysfunction from various organic causes. The men were first tested in the clinic with up to four doses of the drug (125, 250, 500, and 1000µg); those who had sufficient responses were randomly assigned to treatment with either the effective dose of alprostadil or placebo for three months at home.

Results: during in-clinic testing, 996 men (65.9 percent) had erections sufficient for intercourse. Of these men, 961 reported the results of at least one home treatment; 299 of the 461 treated with alprostadil (64.9 percent) had intercourse successfully at least once, as compared with 93 of the 500 who received placebo (18.6 percent, P<0.001). On average, 7 of 10 alprostadil administrations were followed by intercourse in men responsive to treatment. The efficacy of alprostadil was similar regardless of age or the cause of erectile dysfunction, including vascular disease, diabetes, surgery, and trauma (P<0.001 for all comparisons with placebo). The most common side effect was mild penile pain, which occurred after 10.8 percent of alprostadil treatments, but the pain rarely resulted in refusal to continue in the study. Hypotension occurred in the clinic in 3.3 percent of men receiving alprostadil. Hypotension-related symptoms were uncommon at home. No men had priapism or penile fibrosis.

Conclusions: in men with erectile dysfunction, transurethral alprostadil therapy resulted in erection in the clinic and in intercourse at home.

Summary

This study was designed to evaluate a system by which alprostadil (prostaglandin E_1) is delivered transurethrally to treat erectile dysfunction. Alprostadil was delivered transurethrally in a double-blind, placebo-controlled study of 1511 men, aged 27–88 years, who had chronic erectile dysfunction from various organic causes. Men who had sufficient responses to different doses of the drug were randomly assigned to treatment with either the effective dose of alprostadil or placebo for 3 months at home. During in-clinic testing, 996 men (65.9%) had erections sufficient for intercourse. Of these men, 961 reported the results of at least one home treatment; 299 of the 461 treated with alprostadil (64.9%) had successful intercourse at least once, compared with 93 of the 500 who received placebo (18.6%, $p < 0.001$). The most common side effect was mild penile pain, which occurred after 10.8% of alprostadil treatments, but the pain rarely resulted in refusal to continue in the study. Hypotension occurred in the clinic in 3.3% of the men receiving alprostadil. No men had priapism or penile fibrosis.

Citation count	82

Related reference (1)	Williams G, Abbou CC, Amar ET, Desvaux P, Flam TA, Lycklama a Nijeholt GA *et al.* Efficacy and safety of transurethral alprostadil therapy in men with erectile dysfunction. MUSE Study Group. *British Journal of Urology* 1998; **81**: 889–894.

Related reference (2)	Porst H. Transurethral alprostadil with MUSE (medicated urethral system for erection) vs intracavernous alprostadil – a comparative study in 103 patients with erectile dysfunction. *International Journal of Impotence Research* 1997; **9**: 187–192.

Key message

In men with erectile dysfunction, transurethral alprostadil therapy resulted in erections in the clinic and in intercourse at home.

Why it's important

This is a thorough study showing a novel transurethral method for the treatment of erectile dysfunction. The results of this study offered a reasonable rationale for use of a transurethral method to administer PGE_1 in the treatment of impotent men.

Strengths

1. A controlled methodology with a fairly large sample size for the assessment of the efficacy of transurethral administration of PGE_1.
2. Informative results that open the door for further basic and clinical studies using different drugs for transurethral treatment of impotence.

Weaknesses

1. Most of the results were attained after administration in the clinic and the at-home treatment period was not long enough.
2. The efficacy of the treatment was given as 'had intercourse successfully at least once', which leaves the reader to wonder whether the success is consistent.

Relevance

With more refinement of drug manufacture and drug combination, this simple method for administering drugs for erectile dysfunction may be of more interest in the future.

Title

Oral sildenafil in the treatment of erectile dysfunction. Sildenafil Study Group

Authors

Goldstein I, Lue TF, Padma-Nathan H, Rosen RC, Steers WD, Wicker PA

Reference

New England Journal of Medicine 1998; **338**: 1397–12404

Abstract

Background: sildenafil is a potent inhibitor of cyclic guanosine monophosphate specific phospho-diesterase type 5 in the corpus cavernosum and therefore increases the penile response to sexual stimulation. We evaluated the efficacy and safety of sildenafil, administered as needed in two sequential double-blind studies of men with erectile dysfunction of organic, psychogenic, or mixed causes.

Methods: in a 24-week dose-response study, 532 men were treated with oral sildenafil (25, 50 or 100 mg) or placebo. In a 12-week, flexible dose-escalation study, 225 of the 329 men entered a 32-week, open-label extension study. We assessed efficacy according to the International Index of Erectile Function, a patient log, and a global-efficacy question.

Results: in the dose-response study, increasing doses of sildenafil were associated with improved erectile function (P values for increases in scores for questions about achieving and maintaining erections were <0.001). For the men receiving 100 mg of sildenafil, the mean score for the question about achieving erections was 100 percent higher after treatment than at base line (4.0 vs 2.0 of a possible score of 5). In the last four weeks of treatment in the dose-escalation study, 69 percent of all attempts at sexual intercourse were successful for men receiving sildenafil, as compared with 22 percent for those receiving placebo (P<0.001). The mean numbers of successful attempts per month were 5.9 for the men receiving sildenafil and 1.5 for those receiving placebo (P<0.001). Headache, flushing, and dyspepsia were the most common adverse effects in the dose-escalation study occurring in 6 percent to 18 percent of the men. Ninety-two percent of the men completed the 32-week extension study.

Conclusions: oral sildenafil is an effective, well-tolerated treatment for men with erectile dysfunction.

Summary

This study was designed to evaluate the efficacy and safety of oral sildenafil. Results of two sequential double-blind studies of impotent men, who had different organic, psychogenic and mixed causes treated with oral sildenafil, were reported. A statistically significant improvement in the erectile status, as well as successful attempts at intercourse, were achieved in those patients who received sildenafil in comparison to those who received placebo. Headache, flushing and dyspepsia were the most common adverse effects, occurring in 6–18% of men.

Citation count	80

Related reference (1)	Soderling SH, Bayuga SJ, Beavo JA. Identification and characterization of a novel family of cyclic nucleotide phosphodiesterases. *Journal of Biological Chemistry* 1998; **273**: 15553–15538.

Related reference (2)	Ballard SA, Gingell CJ, Tang K, Turner LA, Price ME, Naylor AM. Effects of sildenafil on the relaxation of human corpus cavernosum tissue in vitro and on the activities of cyclic nucleotide phosphodiesterase isozymes. *Journal of Urology* 1998; **159**: 2164–2171.

Related reference (3)	Stief CG, Uckert S, Becker AJ, Truss MC, Jonas U. The effect of the specific phosphodiesterase (PDE) inhibitors on human and rabbit cavernous tissue in vitro and in vivo. *Journal of Urology* 1998; **159**: 1390–1393.

Key message

Oral sildenafil is an effective, well-tolerated treatment for men with erectile dysfunction.

Why it's important

This is a comprehensive study that showed a very promising result to a long-awaited oral treatment of impotence. This study and many consecutive studies have resulted in a resurgence of interest in an oral method of impotence treatment, after a long wait for a successful treatment. Discovery of an effective oral treatment of impotence is well on the way, using more successful oral drugs with fewer adverse effects.

Strengths

1. A well-designed methodology.
2. Clear and readable format.
3. Results are informative and convenient.
4. With more refinement, a life's dream will come true for many patients in the discovery of a 'magic pill', with no side effects, to help impotent men.

Weaknesses

1. Long-term side effects of sildenafil are not yet known.
2. The successful rate in subgroups of patients such as in diabetic, hypertensive etc., was not present.

Relevance

This is a relevant report, demonstrating the efficacy and safety of oral sildenafil for clinical use. This drug has attained increasing popularity; moreover it will be used as a standard for the new emerging oral drugs. It seems unlikely that the release of a single drug could ever again have the same dramatic medical, sociological, political and economic impact as that of sildenafil.

CHAPTER 13

Male infertility

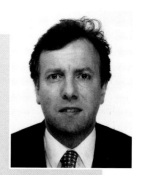

DAVID J RALPH, BSC, MB BS, MS, FRCS(UROL)

- 1980: First degree, BSc in biochemistry, at St Bartholomew's Hospital, London, UK
- 1983: MB BS at St Bartholomew's Hospital, London, UK
- 1996–present: Consultant Urologist at St Peter's Hospital, London, UK
- 1996–present: Honorary Senior Lecturer at Institute of Urology, University College London, UK

Introduction

There have been many classic papers in the field of male infertility in the last 30 years and I have chosen ten papers that I feel represent the classics within individual areas of the field. These have ranged from the understanding of testicular histology from Johnsen, clinical aspects of physiology from Pryor and culminate in the major advances of assisted conception for male infertility by Van Steirteghem. Surgery of male infertility has been addressed, in particular ejaculatory duct obstruction and epididymal obstruction. Contentious issues such as varicocele ligation and antisperm antibody involvement in male infertility have been addressed as has the issue of microsurgical vasovasostomy. Overall, this chapter will give a balanced view of the field of male infertility as it stands today.

Title

Results of 1469 microsurgical vasectomy reversals by the vasovasostomy study group

Authors

Belker AM, Thomas AJ Jr, Fuchs EF, Konnak JW, Sharlip ID

Reference

Journal of Urology 1991; **145**: 505–511

Abstract

During a 9-year period, 1,469 men who underwent microsurgical vasectomy reversal procedures were studied at 5 institutions. Of 1,247 men who had first-time procedures sperm were present in the semen in 865 of 1,012 men (86%) who had post-operative semen analyses, and pregnancy occurred in 421 of 810 couples (52%) for whom information regarding contraception was available. Rates of patency (return of sperm to the semen) and pregnancy varied depending on the interval from the vasectomy until its reversal. If the interval had been less than 3 years, patency was 97% and pregnancy 76%, 3 to 8 years 88% and 53%, 9 to 14 years 79% and 44% and 15 years or more 71% and 30%. The patency and pregnancy rates were no better after 2-layer microsurgical vaso-vasostomy than after modified 1-layer microsurgical procedures and they were statistically the same for all patients regardless of the surgeon. When sperm were absent from the intraoperative vas fluid bilaterally and the patient underwent bilateral vasovasostomy rather than vasoepididymostomy, patency occurred in 50 of 83 patients (60%) and pregnancy in 20 of 65 couples (31%). Neither presence nor absence of a sperm granuloma at the vasectomy site nor type of anesthesia affected results. Repeat microsurgical reversal procedures were less successful. A total of 222 repeat operations produced patency in 150 of 199 patients (75%) who had semen analyses and pregnancy was reported in 52 of 120 couples (43%).

Summary

Microsurgical vasectomy reversal was performed in 1469 men over a 9-year period at five institutions. An overall patency (return of sperm to the semen) rate of 86% and pregnancy rate of 52% was achieved in men having a first-time procedure. A total of 222 repeat operations produced a patency rate of 75% and a pregnancy rate of 43%. The success was significantly associated with the time from the previous vasectomy in that, if the interval had been less than 3 years, the patency rate was 97% and pregnancy 76%, 3–8 years 88% and 53%, 9–14 years 79% and 44%, and at 15 years or more 71% and 30%, respectively. The patency and pregnancy rates were significantly better when the intraoperative findings revealed motile sperm and when the consistency of the vasal fluid was watery rather than creamy in nature. There was no significant difference in the results between the use of a two-layer microsurgical vasovasostomy and a one-layer microsurgical procedure. The results also did not depend on the type of anaesthetic used, whether a granuloma was present at the vasectomy site or the institution assessed.

Citation count   74

Related reference (1)   Silber SJ. Microscopic vasectomy reversal. *Fertility and Sterility* 1977; **28**: 1191–1202.

Related reference (2)   Sharlip ID. Vasovasostomy: comparison of two microsurgical techniques. *Urology* 1981; **17**: 347–352.

Key message

There is no difference in the patency and pregnancy rates between a one- and a two-layer anastomosis. This paper has seen the demise of the latter. Also, the pregnancy and patency rates are dependent on the time interval between the vasectomy and its reversal.

Why it's important

The results of this paper have heralded the demise of the two-layer microsurgical vasovasostomy. Patients can now be given an accurate probable success rate pre-operatively, and can therefore decide whether other assisted conception techniques should be performed together with the reversal of vasectomy. The intraoperative findings, when a thick creamy vasal fluid is obtained in a patient with a long obstructive interval, have now led surgeons to perform elective epididymovasostomies in this situation to improve pregnancy rates.

Strengths

1. A prospective analysis that was multicentre.
2. The paper is now used as a reference to give patients details on the probable success of the operation.
3. Clear answers to questions asked, which have altered andrology practice.

Weaknesses

1. Large number of patients lost to follow-up (approximately 19%).
2. Three institutions performed only a two-layer anastomosis, so the patients were not randomized.

Relevance

The success rates relating to the obstructive interval is used to determine whether simultaneous assisted conception is also necessary. In patients with an obstructive interval of more than 15 years, a low pregnancy rate of 30% has meant that units also either freeze sperm at the time of the reversal or collect fresh sperm using in vitro fertilization and intracytosplamic sperm injection at the time of the reconstruction, to improve pregnancy rates.

Title

Improvement of semen and pregnancy rate after ligation and division of the internal spermatic vein: fact or fiction?

Authors

Nilsson S, Edvinsson A, Nilsson B

Reference

British Journal of Urology 1979; **51**: 591–596

Abstract

Male partners with left-sided varicoceles of **96** infertile couples were studied. Fifty-one patients were submitted to ligation of the testicular veins and **45** individuals were randomised as controls. During an observation period of **53** months (range 36 to 74 months) we found no statistically significant improvement in the semen crude variables, the morphology or the progressive motility in the series of men submitted to surgery. The pregnancy rate was lower in those who had an excision of varicocele.

Summary

This study included 96 couples, with primary unexplained infertility, who had been trying to conceive for at least 2 years. The male partners all had a unilateral left-sided varicocele, which was visible on clinical examination. All patients with a raised level of follicle-stimulating hormone, the presence of antisperm antibodies, azoospermia or a history of previous genital surgery, mumps orchitis or torsion were excluded from the study. All the female partners were shown to be ovulating, 51 patients were submitted to ligation of the testicular veins and 45 individuals were randomized as controls. During a follow-up period of 53 months (range 36–74 months), there was no statistically significant improvement in sperm numbers, motility or morphology. Pregnancy rate was actually lower in those patients who had had ligation of a varicocele.

Citation count	107
Related reference (1)	Dubin L, Amelar RD. Varicocelectomy: 986 cases in a twelve-year study. *Urology* 1977; **10**: 446–449.
Related reference (2)	Tulloch WS. A consideration of sterility factors in the light of subsequent pregnancies: subfertility in the male. *Transactions of the Edinburgh Obstetrics Society* 1952; **59**: 29.

Key message

The first randomized trial to refute the theory that a varicocele is a cause of male infertility.

Why it's important

In 1952, Tulloch (see Related reference (2)) described a varicocelectomy in a patient with bilateral varicoceles and azoospermia. The patient subsequently became normospermic and his wife conceived. Since then there have been many series, notably that of Dubin and Amelar, which reported significant improvements in sperm parameters and pregnancy rates in patients who have varicocele ligation. This paper was one of the first controlled studies that refuted this idea and cast doubt on the association between varicocele and male infertility.

Strengths

1. A prospective, randomized, controlled, clinical trial.
2. A simple study with a clear answer.
3. Partially changed urological practice in that varicoceles are not necessarily ligated routinely.

Weaknesses

1. Female tubal patency was not assessed.
2. Stated that there was no recurrence of varicocele in 51 cases: not investigated and an unexpectedly high success rate in that the recurrence rate is usually up to 20%.

Relevance

For the preceding 25 years, all urologists routinely ligated varicoceles in infertile men; this paper has cast doubt on the value of this procedure and has changed many urologists' view on the association of varicocele with male infertility.

Title

Plasma gonadotrophic hormones, testicular biopsy and seminal analysis in the men of infertile marriages

Authors

Pryor JP, Pugh RCB, Cameron KM, Newton JR, Collins WP

Reference

British Journal of Urology 1976; **48**: 709–717

Abstract

Not available

Summary

Assessment of spermatogenesis in 93 azoospermic and 65 oligozoospermic men was made. The assessment included the testicular size, the plasma levels of follicular-stimulating hormone (FSH) and testicular biopsy at the time of testicular exploration. Spermatogenesis was assessed using the Johnsen scoring method (see Related reference (2)). Testicular size alone was an unreliable means of assessing spermatogenesis because 6% of men with bilateral small testes had normal spermatogenesis on biopsy and 6% of men with normal-sized testes had absent spermatogenesis on biopsy. The plasma FSH level was a reliable guide to the spermatogenesis on testicular biopsy: 29 of 32 patients with a normal FSH had obstructive azoospermia and normal spermatogenesis; grossly elevated FSH levels (more than twice the normal range) were present in 37 and no spermatogenesis or gross impairment of spermatogenesis was present in 36 of these. The paper concludes that testicular exploration and biopsy is unnecessary in azoospermic men with grossly elevated FSH levels and the patients should be advised to consider artificial insemination by donor or adoption.

Citation count	28
Related reference (1)	Pryor JP, Cameron KM, Collins WP, Hirsh AV, Mahony JDH, Pugh RCB, Fitzpatrick JM. Indications for testicular biopsy or exploration in azoospermia. *British Journal of Urology* 1978; **50**: 591–594.
Related reference (2)	Johnsen SG. Testicular biopsy score count: a method for registration of spermatogenesis in human testes: normal values and results in 335 hypogonadal males. *Hormones* 1970; **1**: 2–25.

Key message

The degree of spermatogenesis is inversely proportional to the FSH level. Gross elevation of the FSH level usually signifies the absence of normal spermatogenesis as a cause for azoospermia.

Why it's important

Before the use of plasma FSH levels, spermatogenesis was assessed by testicular biopsy. This paper describes a non-invasive method of assessing spermatogenesis via the plasma FSH level taken together with testicular size. After the 1978 paper by Pryor *et al.* (see Related reference (1)), this led to acceptance that patients with bilateral small testes and grossly elevated FSH levels did not need further investigation because they were likely to have primary testicular failure; therefore they should proceed to either artificial insemination by donor (AID) or adoption. This prevented many men from undergoing unnecessary exploratory operations.

Strengths

1. Clear guidelines given for the management of azoospermia.
2. Demonstrated the importance of FSH estimation in male infertility.

Weaknesses

1. No statistical analysis.
2. Normal values of FSH and testicular size not documented.

Relevance

This paper, together with Related reference (1), established the management of patients with azoospermia. Men with bilateral small testes and grossly elevated FSH levels (more than twice normal) were no longer explored and patients were immediately offered AID or adoption. Patients with FSH levels less than twice normal, or with normal testicular size, continued to have testicular exploration to exclude an obstructive element that could be corrected by reconstruction. This practice is still relevant today, but must not operate in isolation and must be associated with an assisted conception unit.

Title

Ejaculatory duct obstruction in subfertile males: analysis of 87 patients

Authors

Pryor JP, Hendry WF

Reference

Fertility and Sterility 1991; **56**: 725–730

Abstract

Objective: to study the causes, presentation, and treatment of ejaculatory duct obstruction in sub-fertile males.

Design: collaborative retrospective study of clinical experience collected by two urologists over a 15-year period.

Setting: National Health Service and private care hospitals

Patients, participants: subfertile males with azoospermia (n = 67), very severe oligozoospermia (n = 17), oligozoospermia (n = 1) or normal sperm concentration (n = 2) in small volume ejaculates with acid pH and little or no fructose.

Interventions: exploration of scrotum with vasogram and testicular biopsy, plus reconstruction if possible.

Main outcome measures: follow-up seminal analysis and occurrence of pregnancy in female partners.

Results: the causes were: Müllerian duct cyst (n = 17), Wolffian duct malformation (n = 19); previous surgical trauma (e.g. imperforate anus) (n = 15); previous genital infection (n = 19); tuberculosis (n = 8); megavesicles (pathological dilatation of vesicles and ampullae of unknown cause) (n = 8); and carcinoma of prostate (n = 1). After incision of Müllerian duct cysts, five pregnancies were produced. Five pregnancies occurred in the other groups using a variety of surgical techniques.

Conclusions: routine vasography has shown that ejaculatory duct obstruction is not as rare as previously thought. The diagnosis should not be missed because the condition is simple to correct surgically in certain cases.

Summary

The causes and management of 87 patient with ejaculatory duct obstruction are presented. The diagnosis was made via the semen analyses, which was of small volume, acid pH and with little or no fructose; this was deemed pathognomonic in the presence of normal vas deferens. The diagnosis was confirmed by vasography. Sixty-seven patients were azoospermic, 17 with very severe oligozoospermia and two with a normal semen concentration. The causes of ejaculatory duct obstruction were Müllerian duct cyst (17), Wolffian duct malformation (19), traumatic (15), post-infective (19), tuberculosis (eight), megavesicles (eight) and neoplastic (one), totalling 87. The obstruction was amenable to surgery in 31 patients who were treated by transurethral incision/resection. This resulted in patency in 18 patients and six pregnancies were produced.

Citation count   46

Related reference (1) Hendry WF, Pryor JP. Müllerian duct (prostatic utricle) cyst: diagnosis and treatment in subfertile males. *British Journal of Urology* 1992; **69**: 79–82.

Related reference (2) Silber SJ. Ejaculatory duct obstruction. *Journal of Urology* 1980; **124**: 294–297.

Key message

Ejaculatory duct obstruction is not as rare as previously thought and can be a simple condition to correct surgically. Patients with a small-volume ejaculate that has an acid pH and contains little or no fructose should be suspected of having this condition.

Why it's important

There are many causes of ejaculatory duct obstruction, which in itself is a not uncommon cause of azoospermia. Surgical treatment, particularly for Müllerian duct cysts, is simple and can achieve patency in excess of 50%. It is also important to realize that congenital abnormalities at this level may also be associated with renal congenital abnormalities.

Strengths

1. A clear classification of ejaculatory duct obstruction.
2. Beautiful vasography pictures.
3. It shows the importance of a complete semen analysis to include measurement of the volume and pH in all cases, together with fructose when necessary.

Weakness

1. Vague data on post-operative semen analysis.

Relevance

Urologists should be aware of the possible diagnosis of ejaculatory duct obstruction, because this may be an easily treatable condition without the necessity for assisted conception. The importance of a full semen analysis, to include pH, volume and facility to measure fructose, is emphasized.

Title

The role of the human epididymis in sperm maturation and sperm storage as reflected in the consequences of epididymovasostomy

Authors

Schoysman RM, Bedford JM

Reference

Fertility and Sterility 1986; **46**: 293–299

Abstract

Epididymovasostomy has been used for examination of the role of particular regions of the epididymis in sperm maturation and storage, as reflected in fertility and in the motility, structural, and surface character, and also the number of the spermatozoa ejaculated. Human spermatozoa need be exposed only to the environment in the caput before passing into the vas deferens, in order to complete their maturation. However, the chance of pregnancy appears greater where the anastomosis is lower. Among the sperm characteristics examined, only motility was affected by the level of anastomosis, and there was a trend to higher numbers where the anastomosis was established beyond the upper caput. The storage function of the cauda is dismissed in light of the finding that epididymovasostomy patients sometimes ejaculate sperm numbers seen in normal men.

Summary

Epididymovasostomy has been used for examination of particular regions of the epididymis in sperm maturation and storage, as reflected in fertility and in the motility, structural and surface character, and also the number of the spermatozoa ejaculated. This study assesses 117 patients with a successful epididymovasostomy, each with sperm numbers of greater than 20×10^6/ml. Human spermatozoa need be exposed only to the environment in the caput epididymis, before passing into the vas deferens, in order to complete their maturation. However, the chance of pregnancy appears to be greater where the anastomosis is lower. Among the sperm characteristics examined, only motility was affected by the level of anastomosis, and there was a trend to higher numbers where the anastomosis was established beyond the upper caput epididymis, at least 10 mm from the proximal border. The storage function of the cauda epididymis is discussed in light of the finding that epididymovasostomy patients sometimes ejaculate the sperm numbers seen in normal men.

Citation count	46

Related reference (1)	Pryor JP. Surgical opportunities to explore the function of the human epididymis. *Annals of the Royal College of Surgeons of England* 1996; **78**: 49–55.

Key message

When correcting obstructive azoospermia by epididymovasostomy, the anastomosis should be made as low down in the epididymis as possible to allow sperm to mature, and therefore for subsequent increased potential for fertility.

Why it's important

The results give convincing evidence that the anastomosis of epididymovasostomy must be as low as possible to give good pregnancy rates. This is because sperm mature within the epididymis, and will gain progressional motility and hence the greater fertilizing capacity. The data are backed up by Pryor (see Related reference (1)), where the fertilizing capacity of sperm, taken from different regions of the epididymis, with zona free hamster eggs confirmed that the fertilization rate ranged from 0 for sperm from the caput epididymis to 43% for sperm from the cauda epididymis. This was compared with the 68% fertilization rate with ejaculated sperm.

Strengths

1. A large series of patients with known honest reporting of results.
2. Clinical and scientific information incorporated well.
3. An excellent discussion to highlight epididymal function.

Weaknesses

1. Fertility data known on 565 patients, but some of the analyses done on only 35 patients.
2. Negative results of quality/sperm surface investigations.

Relevance

This paper gives a good understanding of the function of the human epididymis and alerts surgeons to perform a low anastomosis during epididymovasostomy, to increase fertilization capacity and pregnancy rate. This is more important in particular when in vitro fertilization and assisted conception are not available.

Title

Testicular obstruction: clinicopathological studies

Authors

Hendry WF, Levinson DA, Parkinson MC, Parslow JM, Royle MG

Reference

Annals of the Royal College of Surgeons of England 1990; **72**: 396–407

Abstract

Genital tract reconstruction has been attempted in subfertile men with obstructive azoospermia (370 patients) or unilateral testicular obstruction (80 patients), and in vasectomised men undergoing reversal for the first time (130 patients) or subsequent (32 patients) time. Histopathological changes in the obstructed testes and epididymes, and immunological responses to the sequestered spermatozoa have been studied to gain insight into possible causes of failure of surgical treatment. The results of surgery have been assessed by follow-up sperm counts and occurrence of pregnancies in the female partners. The best results were obtained with vasectomy reversal (patency 90%, pregnancy 45%), even after failed previous attempts (patency 87%, pregnancy 37%), while postinfective vasal blocks were better corrected by total anatomical reconstruction (patency 73%, pregnancy 27%) than by transvasovasostomy (patency 9%, no pregnancies). Poor results were obtained with capital blocks (patency 12%, pregnancy 3%), in which substantial lipid accumulation was demonstrated in the ductuli efferentes; three-quarters of these patients had sinusitis, bronchitis or bronchiectasis (Young's syndrome). There is circumstantial evidence to suggest that this syndrome may be a late complication of mercury intoxication in childhood.

After successful reconstruction, fertility was relatively reduced in those men who had antibodies to spermatozoa, particularly amongst the postinfective cases. Similarly, impaired fertility was found in men with unilateral testicular obstruction and antibodies to spermatozoa. Mononuclear cell infiltration of seminiferous tubules and rete testis was noted occasionally, supporting a diagnosis of autoimmune orchitis; although rare, this was an important observation as the sperm output became normal with adjuvant prednisolone therapy.

Summary

Genital tract reconstruction was attempted in 370 patients with obstructive azoospermia, 80 patients with unilateral obstruction and 162 patients with a reversal of vasectomy. Histological changes in the obstructed testes and epididymes and the immunological response to the sequestered spermatozoa were studied to gain insight into possible causes of failure of surgical treatment. The results of surgery were assessed by follow-up semen analyses and pregnancies (see Table).

Antisperm antibodies caused by obstruction were measured in most patients. It was found that, after a successful reconstruction, pregnancy was significantly enhanced in the absence of antisperm antibodies. Histological studies showed a mononuclear infiltration to support a diagnosis of autoimmune orchitis, which responded favourably to prednisolone therapy.

	Number	Patency (%)	Pregnancy (%)
Epididymovasostomy (caput)	90	12	3
Epididymovasostomy (cauda)	60	52	38
Post infective vasal reconstruction	11	73	27
Transvasal vasostomy	11	9	0
Vasectomy reversal	130	90	45

Citation count	22

Related reference (1)	Hendry WF, Hughes L, Scammell G, Pryor JP, Hargreave TB. Comparison of prednisolone and placebo in subfertile men with antibodies to spermatozoa. *The Lancet* 1990; **335**: 85–88.

Key message

Testicular obstruction is a common cause of the formation of antisperm antibodies, which may explain the discrepancy between patency and pregnancy rates in all studies after a successful reconstruction.

Why it's important

This paper describes the expected success rates with the different aetiologies of testicular obstruction. Each category is complemented with details of antisperm antibody levels, which may explain why the pregnancy rates are not as high as the patency rates. A placebo-controlled, double-blind, crossover trial of cyclical prednisolone has confirmed that the treatment of antisperm antibodies in this way can improve the pregnancy rate after reconstruction.

Strengths

1. A large number of patients with various types of genital reconstruction.
2. The association of testicular obstruction and antisperm antibody is well documented.
3. Introduces the concept of orchidectomy for the treatment of antisperm antibodies.

Weakness

1. Method of antisperm antibody measurement is controversial.

Relevance

Antisperm antibodies may be caused by testicular obstruction and may persist after successful reconstruction. This may be one reason why pregnancy does not occur after a successful reconstruction and prednisolone therapy can then be instigated.

Title

Is conventional sperm analysis of any use?

Authors

Hargreave TB, Elton RA

Reference

British Journal of Urology 1983; **55**: 774–779

Abstract

The computerised records of 867 couples were used to investigate the prognostic significance of semen volume, motility, density and morphology. The couple-months method of statistical analysis was used, with allowance being made for the duration of involuntary infertility (trying time). Both motility and density were shown to give independent prognostic information, and a table of estimated probabilities is presented which may be helpful when advising the infertile couple on their chances of future conception. If the product of the motility times the density exceeded 0.5 million motile sperm per ml, then one semen analysis was sufficient from the point of view of giving a prognosis.

Summary

The computerized records of 867 couples were used to investigate the prognostic significance of semen volume, motility, density and morphology. The statistical analysis used made allowance for the duration of involuntary infertility (trying time). Both the motility and the density were shown to give independent prognostic information. If the product of the motility and the density exceeded 0.5×10^6 motile sperm/ml, then one semen analysis was sufficient to give the couple a prognosis and a table is presented of the estimated probabilities of conception during the next year, based on the motile sperm concentration and number of months the couple have been trying for pregnancy (see Table).

This table is useful when advising infertile couples on the chances of future conception.

Millions of motile sperm/ml	Trying time (months)			
	12	24	48	96
0	0	0	0	0
0.5	16%	12%	9%	6%
1	25%	19%	14%	9%
2	34%	26%	19%	13%
5	36%	28%	21%	14%
10+	37%	28%	21%	14%

Citation count

37

Related reference (1)

World Health Organization. *WHO Laboratory Manual for the Examination of Human Semen and Sperm Mucous Interaction*, 3rd edn. Cambridge: Cambridge University Press 1992.

Related reference (2)

Macleod J, Gold RZ. The male factor in fertility and infertility. II. Spermatozoon counts in 1000 men of known fertility and in 1000 cases of infertile marriage. *Journal of Urology* 1951; **66**: 436–449.

Key message

The chance of spontaneous conception does not significantly differ once there are more than 2×10^6 motile sperm/ml in the ejaculate. This being so, the worse prognostic indicator is the number of months for which the couple have been trying for a pregnancy.

Why it's important

Oligozoospermia is defined as sperm density of less than 20×10^6/ml, and it is clear that many fertile men have counts much lower than this. This paper therefore emphasizes that motile sperm counts of $2-5 \times 10^6$/ml are adequate for fertility, and that the chance for conception does not change with increasing sperm numbers. The concept of the trying time is introduced in that the longer the couple have been trying to conceive the less likely they are to have spontaneous conception.

Strengths

1. Good statistical analysis.
2. Introduction of trying time.
3. Alerted andrologists that fertility is possible with sperm counts of $2-5 \times 10^6$/ml.

Weakness

1. Statistical calculations often difficult to follow.

Relevance

This paper suggested that a single semen analysis is sufficient to give a prognosis, provided that the motile sperm count is greater than $2-5 \times 10^6$/ml. When also taking the trying time into consideration, clinicians can use the table provided to give advice to patients on the probability of natural conception; this may help in the decision of whether to attempt assisted conception techniques.

Title

The development of intracytoplasmic sperm injection

Authors

Van Steirteghem A, Nagy P, Joris H, Verheyen G, Smitz J, Camus M, Tournaye H, Ubaldi F, Bonduelle M, Silber S, Liebaers I, Devroey P

Reference

Human Reproduction 1996; **11**(suppl 1): 59–72

Abstract

Not available

Summary

This report describes a 4-year survey of 2853 cycles of intracytoplasmic sperm injection (ICSI) in 1953 couples. Ejaculated spermatozoa were used in 91% of the samples, epididymal spermatozoa in 5% and testicular spermatozoa in the remaining 4% of the cycles. In only 7% of the cycles were the ejaculated seminal parameters normal. Overall, 70% of the collected eggs fertilized and 65% of the embryos were transferred. The embryo transfer per cycle was 91% and pregnancy rate per cycle 34% (see Table). The number of embryos transferred per cycle was similar with all types of sperm used, whether it was ejaculated sperm with normal or abnormal semen parameters or epididymal or testicular sperm.

Sperm source	Fertilization rate (%)	Embryo transfer/cycle (%)	Pregnancy/cycle (%)
Ejaculated	71	93	34
Epididymal	58	91	39
Testicular	60	90	36

Citation count   15

Related reference (1)   Van Steirteghem AC, Liu J, Joris H, Nagy Z, Janssenwillen C, Tournaye H *et al.* Higher success rate by intracytoplasmic sperm injection than by subzonal insemination. Report of a second series of 300 consecutive treatment cycles. *Human Reproduction* 1993; **8**: 1055–1060.

Related reference (2)   Steptoe PC, Edwards RG. Birth after the reimplantation of a human embryo. *The Lancet* 1978; **2**(8085): 366.

Related reference (3)   Palermo G, Joris H, Devroey P, Van Steirteghem AC. Pregnancies after intracytoplasmic injection of a single spermatozoon into an oocyte. *The Lancet* 1992; **340**: 17–18.

Key message

The fertilization, embryo transfer and pregnancy rates per cycle of ICSI are similar whether ejaculated sperm of good or poor quality, or epididymal or testicular sperm are used.

Why it's important

After the first birth by in vitro fertilization (IVF) (see Related reference (2)) and then ICSI (see Related reference (3)), it soon became apparent that fertilization using conventional IVF for male factor infertility was poor and that this could be overcome by ICSI. This paper shows that the quality of the sperm is now irrelevant, and fertilization and embryo transfer should occur in over 90% of cycles started.

Strengths

1. Every access of the ICSI programme is discussed in depth.
2. Large numbers give meaningful data.
3. Concentrates mainly on male factor infertility.

Weaknesses

1. Reference biased to own unit.
2. Results relating to aetiology not given.

Relevance

Using ICSI, semen quality is now practically irrelevant with regard to the embryo transfer and pregnancy rates. ICSI has now superseded conventional IVF as the main method of assisted conception for male factor infertility.

Title

Percutaneous epididymal sperm aspiration and intracytoplasmic sperm injection in the management of infertility due to obstructive azoospermia

Authors

Craft I, Tsirigotis M, Bennett V, Taranissi, Khalifa Y, Hogewind G, Nicholson N

Reference

Fertility and Sterility 1995; **65**: 1038–1042

Abstract

Objective: to evaluate the recovery rate of spermatozoa from the epididymis using a percutaneous aspiration technique and to examine the fertilization rate after intracytoplasmic sperm injection.
Design: prospective observational study.
Setting: private infertility clinic, London
Subjects: twenty patients with obstructive azoospermia who each had an attempt at IVF. The sperm used for intracytoplasmic sperm injection was retrieved by percutaneous epididymal sperm aspiration in 16 patients. In one patient, microepididymal sperm aspiration was performed in addition because the quality of the sperm obtained by percutaneous epididymal sperm aspiration was not considered suitable for microinjection. In the remaining three patients, neither percutaneous epididymal sperm aspiration nor microepididymal sperm aspiration resulted in the recovery of sperm, which was obtained by testicular biopsy in one of them.
Intervention: assisted fertilization with intracytoplasmic sperm injection.
Main outcome measures: normal fertilization and pregnancy rates.
Results: a total of 179 eggs were collected and 157 subsequently were microinjected. Normal fertilization occurred in 22 oocytes (14%) and the total number of embryos cleaved was 30. Twelve patients underwent ET in which three conceived (pregnancy rate 25% per transfer). The implantation rate was 10% and failed fertilization occurred in four cycles.
Conclusion: percutaneous epididymal sperm aspiration can be used successfully to recover sperm in men with obstructive azoospermia for use in assisted fertilization in IVF cycles. The technique is simple, effective, and less traumatic compared with an open microsurgical operation.

Summary

Percutaneous epididymal sperm aspiration was performed in 16 patients as the chosen method of sperm retrieval for intracytoplasmic sperm injection (ICSI). All patients had obstructive azoospermia resulting from failed vasectomy reversal (10), congenital absence of the vas deferens (four) or inflammatory obstruction (two). After ICSI, 12 patients underwent embryo transfer and three conceived (pregnancy rate of 25% per embryo transfer).

Citation count	45

Related reference (1)	Silber S, Nagy ZP, Liu J, Godoy H, Devroey P, Van Steirteghem AC. Conventional in vitro fertilisation versus intracytoplasmic sperm injection for patients requiring microsurgical sperm aspiration. *Human Reproduction* 1994; **9**: 1705–1709.
Related reference (2)	Silber SJ, Ord T, Balmaceda J, Patrizio P, Asch R. Congenital absence of the vas deferens. The fertilising capacity of human epididymal sperm. *New England Journal of Medicine* 1990; **323**: 1788–1792.

Key message

Open surgical sperm retrieval is now unnecessary, unless there is a possibility of microsurgical reconstruction being performed concurrently.

Why it's important

This has revolutionized the way in which sperm are retrieved for in vitro fertilization (IVF) and ICSI cycles. Fresh sperm can be harvested on the day by this minimally invasive technique, without the need for coordination of open surgery and egg collection. The procedure can be performed under local anaesthetic and can be repeated.

Strengths

1. A well-written paper describing a simple and new technique.
2. Excellent description of the methods.
3. Describes an outpatient procedure for sperm retrieval.

Weaknesses

1. Does not describe limitations of the technique.
2. Should complement and not replace reconstructive surgery.

Relevance

Percutaneous epididymal sperm aspiration has allowed patients who do not wish to, or are unable to, have obstructive azoospermia corrected by reconstruction the chance to retrieve sperm by this minimally invasive technique. The technique can be repeated to give a source of fresh sperm for IVF and ICSI cycles on the day without the need for open surgical treatment.

Title

Testicular biopsy score count – a method for registration of spermatogenesis in human testes: normal values and results in 335 hypogonadal males

Author

Johnsen SG

Reference

Hormones 1970; **1**: 2–25

Abstract

The paper describes a new and rapid method for registration of spermatogenesis in human testes: the testicular biopsy score count. Each tubular section is given a score from 10 to 1 according to presence or absence of the main cell types arranged in the order of maturity. Presence of spermatozoa scores 10, 9 or 8; spermatids (and no further) 7 or 6; spermatocytes (and no further) 5 or 4; only spermatogonia 3, only Sertoli cells 2 and no cells 1. The theoretical background of the score count method is discussed and it is emphasized that tissue heterogeneity, being a main point in most conditions, is exposed and evaluated by the method.

Normal values are given and results obtained in 335 cases including a great variety of forms of male hypogonadism are presented. Pathognomonic score counts leading to immediate diagnosis at a glance are obtained in many instances. A high correlation between testicular biopsy score count and sperm count is found and it is concluded that by this method it has for the first time become possible in man to correlate endocrine conditions with the functional state of the testicular tissue.

Summary

The testicular biopsy score count is a method of registration of spermatogenesis in the human testes. From a testicular biopsy, each tubular section is given a score from 1 to 10 depending on the absence or presence of the main cell types arranged in the order of maturity. The presence of spermatozoa scores 10, 9 or 8, spermatids 7 or 6, spermatocytes 5 or 4, spermatogonia 3, Sertoli cells only 2 and no cells 1. Many tubular sections are assessed in each biopsy and the tissue is then given a mean Johnsen score. Assessment of 335 patients was made ranging from normal pathology, severe oligozoospermia to azoospermia and in known aetiology groups. There was a high correlation between the Johnsen score and the sperm count ($r = 0.82$; $p < 0.001$).

Citation count	185

Related reference (1)	Tournaye H, Liu J, Nagy PZ, Camus M, Goossens A, Silber S *et al.* Correlation between testicular histology and outcome after intracytoplasmic sperm injection using testicular spermatozoa. *Human Reproduction* 1996; **11**: 127–132.

Related reference (2)   Silber SJ, Nagy Z, Devroey P, Tournaye H, Van Steirteghem AC. Distribution of spermatogenesis in the testicles of azoospermic men: the presence or absence of spermatids in the testes of men with germinal failure. *Human Reproduction* 1997; **12**: 2422–2428.

Key message

An excellent method for registration of spermatogenesis in testicular tissues. The mean score count has guided subsequent management in infertile patients.

Why it's important

The Johnsen score has been used for over 30 years routinely and has given an accurate reflection on the status of spermatogenesis within the testicle. Although there is a high correlation between the Johnsen score and the sperm count, a few normal patients had a low Johnsen score and vice versa. The paper specifies that other areas of testicle may have differing degrees of spermatogenesis. This has been proven as, and testicular sperm can be extracted for ICSI in patients known to have only Sertoli cells with absence of germ cells on a previous biopsy. In one biopsy (see Related reference (1)), the sperm recovery rate was 76% in patients with complete germ-cell aplasia. However, in patients with a high Johnsen score on a previous testis biopsy, sperm are more likely to be extracted during sperm retrieval procedure for ICSI than in patients with germ-cell aplasia (see Related reference (2)).

Strengths

1. Methods well described.
2. Individual Johnsen score counts easy to follow by histopathologists and therefore little variation in reporting by different centres.
3. Histological method still used routinely 28 years later.

Weaknesses

1. Arbitrary figure of total sperm count of 20×10^6 per ml used in classification.
2. No mention of semen analysis in some aetiological groups.
3. Normal patients may not be normal.

Relevance

This is the best method to document spermatogenesis in the testicle. In the patients, it mentions that there may be variations in spermatogenesis in different areas of the testicle. and it has been confirmed that sperm can be retrieved from areas of the testicle where a Johnsen score of 2 has previously been reported.

CHAPTER 14

Stone disease

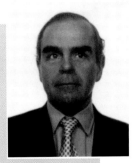

HUGH N WHITFIELD, MA, MCHIR, FRCS, FEBU

- 1969–1974: Short service commission, Royal Army Medical Corps
- 1974–1976: Research Registrar, Institute of Urology, London, UK
- 1976–1979: Registrar, St Bartholomew's Hospital, London, UK
- 1979–1993: Consultant Urologist, St Bartholomew's Hospital, London, UK
- 1980: Hunterian Professor, Royal College of Surgeons of England, London, UK
- 1993–present: Consultant Urologist, Central Middlesex Hospital, London, UK
- 1994: Editor, *British Journal of Urology*, International
- 1996–present: Reader in Urology, Institute of Urology and Nephrology, London, UK
- 1998–present: Civilian Consultant in Urology to the Army
- 1998–2000: President, European Board of *Urology*

Introduction

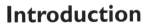

The history of the modern management of urinary tract stone disease spans 30 years. I was involved in the development of intrarenal surgery at the time when preservation of renal function during ischaemia was first introduced. Subsequently, I performed percutaneous renal surgery in the early 1980s. By the mid-1980s, these challenging techniques had been established as routine surgical procedures. In 1985, the first Dornier lithotripter came to the United Kingdom, and I had the opportunity to use it on a regular basis. Subsequent developments both in extracorporeal lithotripsy and in ureteric endoscopy have continued to reduce the morbidity of stone disease. I have picked papers that represent the most important milestones in the development of current management of stones. Many urologists in training tend to ignore literature that is more than 10 years old; they do so at their peril. The collection of papers that I have made maps what has been little short of a revolution, and I hope has helped to provoke ideas for future studies that need to be done. By including a paper on the metabolic aspects of stone disease, I wish to stress the importance of providing, in a stone centre, a comprehensive range of medical and surgical investigations and treatment.

Title

The anatomy of the intrarenal arteries and its application to segmental resection of the kidney

Author

Graves FT

Reference

British Journal of Surgery 1954; **42**: 132–9

Abstract

Not available

Summary

The author used two methods of investigating kidneys removed *post mortem*. Polyester resin was injected into the renal artery and the kidney substance was subsequently removed with hydrochloric acid. Angiography and venography of postmortem specimens were also performed. He showed that the kidney could be divided into five segments: apical, upper anterior, middle anterior, lower and posterior. Each segment was supplied by its own artery. The main stem of the artery divided at a variable point between the aorta and the renal hilum into an anterior and posterior division. The anterior division gave rise to the upper, middle and lower segmental arteries, and the apical segment artery usually also arose from it. The posterior division supplied only the posterior segment but on occasions could give rise to the apical segment artery.

Citation count	57
Related reference (1)	Graves FT. *Anatomical Studies for Renal and Intrarenal Surgery*. Bristol: Wright, 1986.
Related reference (2)	Brodel M. The intrinsic blood-vessels of the kidney and their significance in nephrotomy. *Bulletin of the Johns Hopkins Hospital* 1901; **12**: 10–13.
Related reference (3)	Boyce WH. Anatrophic nephrotomy. In: *Intra-renal Surgery* (Wickham JEA, ed.). London: Churchill Livingstone, 1984: Chapter 7.

Key message

The observations in this study showed that segmental arteries are end arteries and that conservative renal surgery must be performed in the light of this anatomy.

Why it's important

When this study was performed initially, surgeons were just beginning to recognize the possibility of conservative renal surgery for renal tuberculosis and renal calculus disease. The knowledge of the vascular anatomy of the kidney was incomplete and this study defined the arterial distribution within the kidney. Graves showed that, although there were variations, the basic pattern of distribution was quite standard, and he defined five main segments. He also identified the fact that there was no anastomosis between the arterial supply of different segments. He showed that the venous systems freely anastomosed within the kidney. He discussed the significance of these anatomical findings in relation to surgical practice.

Strengths

1. The author showed that Brodel's 'bloodless line' (see Related reference (2)) does not exist.
2. The anatomy that is defined is of relevance to open surgery and to percutaneous renal surgery.
3. The paper advocated pre-operative renal arteriography to help plan conservative renal surgery.
4. It identified that segmental arteries were end arteries.
5. It identified the concentration of veins posterior to a calyx.

Weaknesses

1. This was an in vitro study using casts of the kidney produced either by injected coloured resins or by arteriography.
2. There were no corroborative functional studies performed on an in vivo model.

Relevance

Conservative renal surgery for stone disease and for malignant disease remains an important aspect of urological surgery. A knowledge of renal vascular anatomy is equally important when performing percutaneous renal surgery. These studies showed the way forward in the understanding of how such surgery could be performed most safely.

Title

Bilateral renal calculi

Authors

Sreenevasan G

Reference

Annals of the Royal College of Surgeons of England 1974; **55**: 3–12

Abstract

Bilateral renal calculi were present in 114 (10.7%) of 1,070 cases of proved urinary calculus admitted to the Urological Department of the General Hospital, Kuala Lumpur, during the period November 1968–May 1973. The management of bilateral renal calculi is discussed with reference to the first 100 cases in this series. The introduction of renography has greatly facilitated the decision as to which kidney should be operated on first. The management of patients with and without uraemia is discussed and the use of the modified V and V-Y incisions for the removal of staghorn calculi is described. Complications and results are briefly reviewed.

Summary

One hundred and fourteen patients with bilateral renal calculi were studied between 1968 and 1973. During this time renography was introduced. They also showed that the criteria suggested by Farquharson and Aird were flawed and they quote two case histories to support this. They continued by reporting a case in whom renography was used to determine correctly which side to operate on first. Based on clinical experience, guidelines were established. Follow-up of these patients proved the value of this approach.

Citation count	4
Related reference (1)	Holm-Nielsen A, Jørgensen T, Mogensen P, Fogh J. The prognostic value of probe renography in ureteric stone obstruction. *British Journal of Urology* 1981; **53**: 504–507.
Related reference (2)	Britton KE, Brown NJG. *Clinical Renography.* London: Lloyd-Luke 1971: 141–171.
Related reference (3)	Whitfield HN, Britton KE, Nimmon CC, Hendry WF, Wallace DM, Wickham JE. Renal transit time measurements in the diagnosis of ureteric obstruction. *British Journal of Urology* 1981; **53**: 500–503.
Related reference (4)	Farquharson EL. *Textbook of Operative Surgery*, 2nd edn., Livingstone, Edinburgh 1962: 289
Related reference (5)	Aird I. *A Comparison in Surgical Studies.* Livingstone, Edinburgh 1958.

Key message

Renography alone can accurately define the percentage contribution of each kidney to overall renal function.

Why it's important

This study was the first to compare the management of bilateral renal calculi with and without renography. Previously, the criteria for deciding on which side to operate on first had been suggested by Farquharson (see Related reference (4)) and Aird (see Related reference (5)); they suggested that if a kidney was enlarged this was likely to be the result of hydronephrosis, and that the other kidney should be operated on first. The author showed that these criteria were inappropriate with the use of isotope renography, which was sometimes performed on an emergency basis. In his overall series of 1070 cases, he focused on 100 patients with bilateral stone disease. He showed that it was important to operate on the better kidney first. He stressed the importance of rehydrating a patient, particularly those with uraemia, pre-operatively. He also advocated pre-operative haemodialysis in patients with severe renal impairment.

Strengths

1. The paper redefined the criteria for deciding which kidney should be operated on first in cases of bilateral stone disease.
2. It showed that renography can provide reliable results in patients with impaired renal function.
3. It stressed the poor outcome in patients whose bilateral stone disease was left untreated.
4. It advocated the extracapsular approach of Gil-Vernet (fifth paper in this chapter) to the renal sinus, but preferred a 'V'-shaped incision in the pelvis which could be modified into a 'Y' for correction of pelvicoureteral junction narrowing. This avoids the potential devascularization of the renal pelvis which can occur after the standard Gil-Vernet transverse pyelotomy incision.
5. It stressed the potential for recovery in a kidney after stone removal, but recognized that the potential for recovery could not be assessed in any way other than by removing the stone.

Weakness

1. No long-term follow-up renographic studies were reported.

Relevance

This is a classic paper because it shows that individual renal function can only be assessed accurately isotopically and not clinically or by intravenous urography.

Title

Regional renal hypothermia

Authors

Wickham JEA, Hanley HG, Joekes AM

Reference

British Journal of Urology 1967; **39**: 727–743

Abstract

Not available

Summary

The authors begin by reviewing the literature available at that time, related to the period of renal ischaemia that could be tolerated without evidence histologically or physiologically of renal damage. They concluded that there was no consensus view. They undertook a study in rabbits and divided the animals into three groups. In the first, they determined the duration of ischaemia that would produce severe depression of function. In the second, they investigated ways of mitigating the renal damage by varying degrees of renal cooling. In the third, they determined the period of time for which the ischaemic rabbit kidney could be maintained at a temperature of 20°C. On the basis of their experiments, they identified that, in the rabbit kidney, a 3-hour period of ischaemia could be safely maintained if the temperature of the kidney was lowered to 20°C.

Citation count	58
Related reference (1)	Wickham JEA, Fernando AR, Hendry WF, Watkinson LE, Whitfield HN, Armstrong DGM, Griffiths JR. Inosine in preserving renal function during ischaemic renal surgery. *British Medical Journal* 1978; **2**: 173–174.
Related reference (2)	Fernando AR, Armstrong DMG, Griffiths JR, Hendry WF, O'Donoghue EPN, Watkins LE *et al.* Renal function after warm ischaemia. *European Urology* 1977; **3**: 355–358.

Key message

The authors identified the optimal temperature to which the kidney should be lowered for sustaining renal function during a period of renal ischaemia. At 20°C, 3 hours of ischaemia was safe in their experimental model.

Why it's important

This study investigated the benefits of regional renal hypothermia during periods of renal circulatory rest, to allow complex intrarenal surgery to be performed in a dry kidney. Previous studies had shown that ischaemic damage occurred after 30 minutes of arterial arrest. The authors recommended that, to avoid even minimum depression of function, warm ischaemia times should not exceed 10 minutes. Using a rabbit model in vivo, the effect of lowering the renal temperature to different levels was collated with the functional depression that occurred after varying lengths of renal artery occlusion. They showed that it was unnecessary to cool the kidney by intravascular perfusion. They designed a small cooling system, which was subsequently modified for clinical use.

Strengths

1. This paper identified the optimum temperature for cooling the kidney to preserve renal function during ischaemia.
2. This was a well-designed experimental study in a rabbit model.
3. The authors designed a simple apparatus for cooling the kidney externally.
4. The apparatus was cheap and safe.
5. The human studies showed that complete stone clearance is the essential step to sterilizing the urine in patients with stones that are infective in origin.
6. Renal arterial occlusion for complex intrarenal surgery minimizes blood loss.

Weaknesses

1. In this study, no long-term follow-up results of the clinical cases are provided, although, in subsequent papers, Wickham addressed this issue (see Related reference (1)).
2. The experimental study was done in a rabbit model, which has a very different kind of kidney from a human multi-calyceal system. Ideally, the study should have been done in mini-pigs, but the expense of this would have been prohibitive.

Relevance

Whatever the indication for conservative renal surgery, the importance of preserving renal function during periods of renal ischaemia remains of paramount importance. It is more difficult now to obtain the disposables for the Wickham cooling apparatus and most surgeons have to rely on crushed ice. This represents a retrograde step over the way in which such surgery was performed 20 years ago. Nevertheless, the principle of renal cooling during periods of ischaemia in excess of 30 minutes remains a fundamental part of any such technique.

Title

Percutaneous pyelolithotomy: a new extraction technique

Authors

Fernström I, Johansson B

Reference

Scandinavian Journal of Urology and Nephrology 1976; **10**: 257–259

Abstract

Not available

Summary

The authors report three cases in whom they performed an elective dilatation of a nephrostomy track before stone removal that was under radiological control.

Citation count	147

Related reference (1) Whitfield HN. Percutaneous nephrolithotomy. *British Journal of Urology* 1983; **55**: 609–612.

Related reference (2) Alken P. Percutaneous ultrasonic destruction of renal calculi. *Urologic Clinics of North America* 1982; **9**: 145–151.

Related reference (3) Günther R, Altwein JE. Perkutane transrenale Extraktion eines abgerissenen Nephrostomie – Katheters. *Fortschritte auf dem Gebiete der Röntgenstrahlen und der Nuklearmedizin* 1979; **130**: 121–122.

Key message

Elective dilatation of a nephrostomy track before percutaneous stone removal is a practical proposition.

Why it's important

This is the first paper in which a percutaneous tract to the kidney was formed for the specific purpose of subsequently removing an intrarenal stone. Previous reports of percutaneous inspection of the kidney had described using a nephrostomy track inserted at the time of an open operation. These authors, one a radiologist and the other a urologist, showed how the percutaneous approach to the kidney could be performed safely, with the track being dilated under biplanar radiological guidance. In this report. the authors dilated the track progressively over several days, exchanging a slightly larger diameter catheter on each occasion until the track was large enough for removal of the stone by means of a Dormia basket. No anaesthetic was used for changing the catheters, although the stone removal itself was performed under general anaesthesia. At that time, the Amplatz sheath had not been invented and therefore after the last dilatation the track was left to mature for 5–20 days. This paper set the scene for the subsequent development of percutaneous renal surgery.

Strengths

1. This case series of three patients showed that it was safe to dilate a track into the collecting system through the parenchyma, and that such dilatation could be performed under local anaesthesia.
2. Stones up to 15 mm in diameter could be removed without the need for prior disintegration.

Weaknesses

1. No previous animal study had been performed.
2. No pre- or post-operative renal functional study was performed.

Relevance

This paper showed that a technique first described for the use of removing retained common bile duct stones could be applied equally effectively to the kidney. The authors demonstrated a technique that was subsequently rapidly taken up by centres all over the world. The speed of this adoption provides evidence of its effectiveness, although severe critics would say that no randomized, prospective, controlled study was performed. It is doubtful whether any such trial would have been passed by an ethical committee.

Title

New surgical concepts in removing renal calculi

Author

Gil-Vernet J

Reference

Urology International 1965; **20**: 255–288

Abstract

After a critical study of the methods in use for the lithiasis surgery of the kidney the great risk of some of them the inefficacy and the danger – especially in the staghorn cases, the calyceal stones or those contained in a pelvis of intrarenal type – are pointed out. The causes due to the operative lithogenic disease are analysed.

The submitted new surgery for the renal lithiasis is based upon the combined and simultaneous utilization of several principles – some known, such as the surgery of the kidney 'in situ', others modified, such as the posterior vertical lumbotomy replacing the classic and dangerous oblique lumbotomy, and finally some new ones, such as the extracapsular approach to the renal sinus, the transverse intrasinusal pyelotomy incision and the selective calicotomy incision.

The exposure of the renal sinus by this new extracapsular approach is technically easy and offers visibility to all the intrarenal portion of the pelvis and to the major calices. It is completely bloodless.

For several reasons the transverse intrasinusal pyelotomy is far superior to the classic vertical pyelotomy.

The intrasinusal calicolithotomy is also a new term which must enter into the nomenclature and practice of urological surgery. The post-operative stage elapses with no leakage of urine so that drainage of the lumbar fossa is omitted thus avoiding complications. Patients leave the hospital by the seventh and many by the fourth day after the operation.

This type of surgery has changed the prognosis for staghorn calculi and multiple calculi cases obtaining a total extraction with no injury to the renal parenchyma, and no trauma to the excretory tract. It is of great advantage to the patient who carries a simple pelvic calculus.

Following this kind of operation reinterventions do not offer inconveniences, but then, the sinusal space must be entered by way of another approach, the intracapsular one. The number of resources is notoriously lower than those observed with the classic techniques.

Our conclusions are based on an experience of 324 cases of no mortality, no complications and with excellent results.

Summary

This is in the nature of a review paper, in which the author takes a critical look at the ways in which open renal surgery for stone disease were currently being practised. He then proposes new approaches, in particular the transverse intrasinusal pyelotomy, in which the renal pelvis and calyceal infundibula are exposed to give access to most of the intrarenal collecting system.

Citation count	106

Related reference (1)	Boyce WH. Renal calculi. In: *Urological Surgery*, 2nd edn (Glenn JF, ed.). Hagerstown: Harper & Row, 1975: 169–189.

| **Related reference (2)** | Wickham JEA (ed.). The surgical treatment of renal lithiasis. In: *Urinary Calculus Disease*. Edinburgh: Churchill Livingstone, 1979: 145–198. |

Key message

The author identifies a surgical approach to the renal collecting system, which causes minimal renal damage and offers good exposure to the interior of the kidney.

Why it's important

This paper described two aspects of conservative renal surgery for stones. First, the author stressed the morbidity of the classic loin incision to the kidney and recommended a vertical lumbotomy that was muscle splitting rather than muscle cutting. Second, he showed that, by what he described as an 'extracapsular approach' to the renal sinus, it was possible to gain wide exposure of the peripheral collecting system within the kidney, without damaging the posterior branch of the renal artery. He defined the relationship between the renal sinus and the vessels, calyces and renal pelvis. He went on to describe the pyelocalyceal incision for the removal of a complete staghorn stone. He also demonstrated the use of a calicotomy performed within the renal sinus. He stressed the importance of a peroperative radiograph to ensure that complete stone clearance had been achieved.

Strengths

1. The beginning of minimally invasive surgery was recommended, with a vertical lumbotomy incision.
2. Access to the collecting system was described without the need for renal ischaemia.
3. The importance of peroperative radiographs was stressed.
4. Specialized instrumentation was designed to maximize exposure within the renal sinus.
5. The relationship of the collecting system to the vascular anatomy was identified.

Weakness

1. In the summary at the beginning of the paper, the author talks about an experience of 324 cases. The value of his new subcapsular intrarenal sinus approach was, however, really confined to the 19 patients who underwent surgery for staghorn stones.

Relevance

The sinus approach remains a basic technique for conservative renal surgery for stone disease. Although the indications for open renal surgery have diminished since the advent of percutaneous renal surgery and extracorporeal shockwave lithotripsy, there remains a small minority of patients for whom open renal surgery for stones is the method of choice. Surgeons performing such surgery would need to be confident with this surgical approach.

Title

Percutaneous stone manipulation

Authors

Alken P, Hutschenreiter G, Günther R, Marberger M

Reference

Journal of Urology 1981; **125**: 463–466

Abstract

Percutaneous stone manipulation by direct ultrasound disintegration, extraction or chemolysis was done on 34 patients. A total of 15 patients presented with an operatively established nephrostomy, while percutaneous nephrostomy and subsequent dilation of the nephrostomy channel were done in 19. The rate of complete stone clearance was 19 of 20 stones after percutaneous nephrostomy and 8 of 16 stones in the group with an operatively established nephrostomy. The primary goal, to remove obstructing pelvic stones, was achieved in all cases. There were no untoward side effects, such as back pressure damage owing to flushing of the collecting system during ultrasound disintegration, or persistent infection. Complications in 3 patients were managed conservatively.

Summary

The authors describe 34 patients in whom stones were disintegrated or dissolved. In 15 patients the nephrostomy track had been established operatively, and in the remainder an elective percutaneous nephrostomy track had been created. They achieved complete stone clearance in 19 of 20 stones after percutaneous nephrostomy electively, and in 8 of 16 stones in the patients in whom the nephrostomy track had been established at the time of open operation. No significant complications were recorded.

Citation count	147
Related reference (1)	Goodwin WE, Casey WC, Woolf W. Percutaneous trocar (needle) nephrostomy in hydronephrosis. *Journal of the American Medical Association* 1955; **157**: 891.
Related reference (2)	Rupel E, Brown R. Nephroscopy with removal of stone following nephrostomy for obstructive calculous anuria. *Journal of Urology* 1941; **46**: 177.
Related reference (3)	Kurth KH, Hohenfellner R, Altwein JE. Ultrasound litholapaxy of a staghorn calculus. *Journal of Urology* 1977; **117**: 242.

Key message

Elective percutaneous nephrostomy provides the possibility of more complete stone clearance than using a nephrostomy track established at open operation. Stones too large to be removed through the nephrostomy track can be disintegrated or dissolved before removal.

Why it's important

This paper is important for two reasons. First, the authors distinguish between a nephrostomy track that originated after open surgery from a nephrostomy track that was fashioned for the purpose of stone removal. Second, this is the first paper in which methods of stone disintegration are described, allowing stones that are too large to be removed through a nephrostomy channel. The Department of Urology and Radiology at the University of Mainz deserves recognition as the department that popularized percutaneous renal surgery.

Strengths

1. This paper shows the feasibility of disintegrating renal stones before removal, using either ultrasound or an electrohydraulic lithotrite.
2. The safety of the procedure was established.
3. The success of the procedure was established, with complete stone clearance being achieved in 19 of 20 patients in whom a percutaneous nephrostomy track was inserted electively.

Weakness

1. A small case series.

Relevance

This paper is a keystone in percutaneous renal surgery because the technique that they describe was shown to be applicable to a variety of stone types, not just small renal pelvic stones. The fact that some of their patients were operated on for definitive stone removal without any kind of anaesthesia is a tribute to the patients under their care, many of whom were in a high-risk category for one reason or another.

Title

Extracorporeally induced destruction of kidney stones by shock waves

Authors

Chaussy Ch, Brendel W, Schmiedt E

Reference

The Lancet 1980; **II**: 1265–1268

Abstract

High-energy shock waves were used to disintegrate kidney stones in dogs and man. In 96% of 60 dogs with surgically implanted renal pelvic stones, the fragments were discharged in the urine. The same effect was achieved in 20 out of 21 patients with renal pelvic stones. In the twenty-first patient, a staghorn calculus was broken up to facilitate surgical removal. 2 patients with upper ureteric stones also received shock waves, but their stones had to be removed surgically; in 1 of these the stone had been embedded in the ureteric wall by connective tissue. The procedure can in many cases be done under epidural instead of general anaesthesia. Side-effects consisted of slight haematuria and, occasionally, of easily treatable ureteric colic. They were probably due to passage of fragments down the ureter. Disintegration of kidney stones by shock waves seems to be a promising form of treatment that reduces the need for surgery.

Summary

The authors describe the use of high-energy shock waves in disintegrating stones in an animal model and in humans. Renal pelvic stones were implanted into 60 dogs and a 96% fragmentation rate was achieved. In 20 of 21 patients with renal pelvic stones, satisfactory fragmentation was also achieved. Minimal side effects and complications were encountered.

Citation count	314
Related reference (1)	Chaussy Ch, Eisenberger F, Wanner K. The use of shock waves for the destruction of renal calculi without direct contact. *Urological Research* 1976; **4**: 175.
Related reference (2)	Chaussy Ch, Schmiedt E, Forssmann B, Brendel W. Contact-free renal stone destruction by means of shock waves. *European Surgical Research* 1979; **11**: 36.
Related reference (3)	Forssmann B, Hepp W, Chaussy Ch, Eisenberger F, Wanner K. Eine Methode zur berührungsfreien Zertrümmerung von Nierensteinen mit Stosswellen. *Biomedizinische Technik* 1977; **22**: 164.

Key message

Shockwaves induced extracorporeally were shown to disintegrate renal pelvic stones effectively and safely.

Why it's important

This is not the first paper in which the use of extracorporeally induced shock waves for the destruction of kidney stones is described. However, it is the first paper to appear in any major international journal that is aimed at a wide medical and surgical audience. Extracorporeal shock wave lithoptripsy (ESWL) has provoked a revolution in the management of upper urinary tract stones and there are few if any innovations in medicine or surgery at any time in history that merit the same accolade. ESWL could be performed as a day case procedure, albeit under general or epidural anaesthesia initially, and this was replacing a major open surgical operation which required about 7 days in hospital. The impact of this technology was not confined to urology, but later spread to the treatment of cholelithiasis and recently to soft tissue calcification at various sites.

Strengths

1. Earlier experimental studies had shown the safety of the technique.
2. The paper reports the first 21 patients who were treated, beginning in February 1980.
3. The technique was successful in 20 of 21 patients.
4. The authors make cautiously optimistic assessments for the potential of the technique.

Weaknesses

1. Insufficient credit is given to Eisenberger *et al.* (See Related reference (1)) who did much of the original experimental work.
2. The method described, by which the shock wave disintegrates the stone, is speculative and has subsequently been proved wrong.

Relevance

This is a landmark paper, describing a revolution in the management of upper urinary tract stone disease, which has brought benefit to hundreds of thousands of patients world wide. Those who developed this technique might even be in line for a Nobel prize, which would be only the second in urology.

Title

Ureteral and renal endoscopy, a new approach

Authors

Pérez-Castro Ellendt E, Martinez-Piñeiro JA

Reference

European Urology 1982; **8**: 117–120

Abstract

The development of a new rigid instrument for the exploration and treatment of pathologies localized above the ureteral orifice broadens importantly the field of urologic endoscopy. Heretofore, we have used this instrument in 12 patients for the study of various ureteral or renal pathologies. Its advantages over the flexible fiber optic ureteroscope and over the previous timid attempts of ureteroscopy or intraurethral litholapaxy with infantile cystoscopes are obvious. The operative possibilities of this instrument shall change the therapeutic approach to many upper urinary tract conditions.

Summary

The authors describe a ureteronephroscope that they designed and which was manufactured by the Storz company. The instrument was 50 cm long with a 4 French gauge channel for instrumentation. They recommended prior ureteric dilatation if the ureter was not dilated. Alternatively, an indwelling ureteric catheter could be left after the endoscopic procedure to ensure drainage. They report on 12 cases in whom the instrument was used successfully.

Citation count	32

Related reference (1)	Lyon ES, Kyker SJ, Schoemberg HW. Transurethral ureteroscopy in women. A ready addition to the urological armamentarium. *Journal of Urology* 1978; **119**: 35.
Related reference (2)	Lyon ES, Banno JJ, Schoemberg HW. Transurethral ureteroscopy in men using juvenile cystoscopy equipment. *Journal of Urology* 1979; **122**: 152.
Related reference (3)	Das S. Transurethral ureteroscopy and stone manipulation under direct vision. *Journal of Urology* 1981; **125**: 112.

Key message

Ureteroscopy with a rigid endoscope was shown to be safe and effective throughout the length of the ureter.

Why it's important

These authors were the first to describe the use of a new rigid instrument to inspect the whole of the upper urinary tract. Although authors had previously described the use of small-calibre cysto-scopes to inspect the lower part of the ureter, Pérez-Castro Ellendt was the first to demonstrate that the whole of the ureter and part of the intrarenal collecting system could be inspected with a rigid instrument, 50 cm long. He recommended that, if the ureter were of normal calibre, a previous dilatation with ureteric probes should be performed or an indwelling ureteric catheter should be left for 24 hours to facilitate endoscopy.

Strengths

1. The authors warn against using an irrigating pressure that is too high.
2. The potential for operating through the ureterorenoscope was realized, and the possibility of taking ureteric biopsies and removing ureteric tumours and for removing small calculi was reported.
3. The authors made an imaginative speculation about the diagnostic and therapeutic advantages of this technique.
4. The authors identified the fact that the technique was safe, straightforward, economical and accurate.

Weakness

1. The authors felt that the possibility of ureteric perforation was remote, and they believe that 'in the hands of skilled endoscopists the rate of complication should be fairly low'.

Relevance

The use of ureteroscopy has now become standard and the development of improved instrumentation has enhanced the advantages of the technique, which was first described, using a purpose-built instrument, in 1982.

Title

The prognostic value of probe renography in ureteric stone obstruction

Authors

Holm-Nielsen A, Jørgensen T, Mogensen P, Fogh J

Reference

British Journal of Urology 1981; **53**: 504–507

Abstract

During a 4-year period 143 patients were monitored with probe renography during and after obstruction. Cases with obstruction of short duration (less than 2 weeks) all did well. In cases with longer duration the renographic function values could be used to predict irreversible kidney damage. Stone size showed no correlation with functional impairment. Infection proximal to ureteric stones accelerated kidney damage. Recommendations for the control of ureteric stone patients are given.

Summary

The authors studied 239 patients admitted over a 4-year period between 1976 and 1980 with unilateral ureteric stones. In 143 patients, renography had been performed soon after presentation and then subsequently. Seventy-four patients were found to have impaired function during obstruction and they were divided into three groups: those with an obstruction for less than 14 days, those with an obstruction for between 15 and 28 days, and those with an obstruction for more than 28 days. Function returned to normal, after stone treatment, in all patients in whom the obstruction was relieved within 14 days (26 patients). In the second group of 17 patients, obstructed for between 15 and 28 days, renal function returned to normal in 14 of 17 patients. In the last group of 31 patients, 11 showed irreversible renal damage after the relief of obstruction.

Citation count	5

Related reference (1)	Mogensen P, Bay-Nielsen H, Egebald M, Munck O. I-hippuran renography for control of patients with ureterolithiasis. *Scandinavian Journal of Urology and Nephrology* 1976; **10**: 253–256.

Related reference (2)	Britton KE, Brown NJG. *Clinical Renography*. London: Lloyd-Luke, 1971: 141–171.

Related reference (3)	Marshall RH, White RH, Chaput de Saintonge M, Saintonge MC, Tresidder GC, Blandy JP. The natural history of renal and ureteric calculi. *British Journal of Urology* 1975; **47**: 117–124.

Key message

Prolonged ureteric obstruction even in the absence of infection can cause irreversible renal damage.

Why it's important

This paper looked at data on 239 patients presenting acutely with unilateral ureteric stones. In 96 cases the stone passed before renography could be performed. In 143 patients there were renographic data available soon after the patient presented and follow-up data subsequently. These patients showed that there was no connection between the size of the stone and functional impairment. The study also provided data about the accelerated damage occurring when infection was present proximal to a ureteric stone. All patients in whom the duration of obstruction was less than 2 weeks had a return of renal function to normal. Three of 17 patients were obstructed for between 2 and 4 weeks, and 11 of 31 patients with a longer duration of obstruction had irreversible kidney damage. In addition, the authors had some evidence that patients in younger age groups showed greater potential for recovery than more elderly patients, but the numbers were too small to apply this kind of analysis.

Strengths

1. The authors show that symptoms do not correlate with loss of function.
2. They show that the size of the stone is not correlated with the potential for irreversible renal damage.
3. They have shown that there is no way to predict which patients are most at risk.
4. They confirm that infection plus obstruction leads to severe irreversible functional loss.

Weaknesses

1. The size of the whole group and of the subgroups is relatively small.
2. This was a retrospective study.
3. The younger patients with functional impairment were subjected to a more active treatment than elderly patients.

Relevance

This paper shows that, if patients with ureteric stones are to be treated conservatively for more than 2 weeks, careful renographic follow-up is mandatory. This is an important clinical lesson that is still often ignored.

Title

A prospective study of dietary calcium and other nutrients and the risk of symptomatic kidney stones

Authors

Curhan GC, Willett WC, Rimm EB, Stampfer MJ

Reference

New England Journal of Medicine 1993; **328**: 833–838

Abstract

A high dietary calcium intake is strongly suspected of increasing the risk of kidney stones. However, a high intake of calcium can reduce the urinary excretion of oxalate, which is thought to lower the risk. The concept that a higher dietary calcium intake increases the risk of kidney stones therefore requires examination.

Methods: we conducted a prospective study of the relation between dietary calcium intake and the risk of symptomatic kidney stones in a cohort of 45,619 men, 40 to 75 years of age, who had no history of kidney stones. Dietary calcium was measured by means of a semiquantitative food-frequency questionnaire in 1986. During four years of follow-up, 505 cases of kidney stones were documented.

Results: after adjustment for age, dietary calcium intake was inversely associated with the risk of kidney stones; the relative risk of kidney stones for men in the highest as compared with the lowest quintile group for calcium intake was 0.56 (95 per cent confidence interval, 0.43 to 0.73; P for trend, <0.001). This reduction in risk decreased only slightly (relative risk, 0.66; 95 per cent confidence interval, 0.49 to 0.90) after further adjustment for other potential risk factors, including alcohol consumption and dietary intake of animal protein, potassium, and fluid. Intake of animal protein was directly associated with the risk of stone formation (relative risk for men with the highest intake as compared with those with the lowest, 1.33; 95 per cent confidence interval, 1.00 to 1.77); potassium intake (relative risk, 0.49; 95 per cent confidence interval, 0.35 to 0.68) and fluid intake (relative risk, 0.71; 95 per cent confidence interval, 0.52 to 0.97) were inversely related to the risk of kidney stones.

Conclusions: a high dietary calcium intake decreases the risk of symptomatic kidney stones.

Summary

The authors conducted a prospective study in 45 619 men aged between 40 and 75 years who had no history of renal stones. These patients were followed for 4 years, during which time 505 patients developed a renal stone. They identified, after adjustment for age, that dietary calcium intake was inversely associated with the risk of renal stones.

Citation count   155

Related reference (1)   Johnson CM, Wilson DM, O'Fallon WM, Malek RS, Kurland LT. Renal stone epidemiology: a 25-year study in Rochester, Minnesota. *Kidney International* 1979; **16**: 624–631.

| Related reference (2) | Marshall RW, Cochran M, Hodgkinson A. Relationships between calcium and oxalic acid intake in the diet and their excretion in the urine of normal and renal-stone-forming subjects. *Clinical Science* 1972; **43**: 91–99. |
| Related reference (3) | Robertson WG, Peacock M, Hodgkinson A. Dietary changes and the incidence of urinary calculi in the UK between 1958 and 1976. *Journal of Chronic Disease* 1979; **32**: 469–476. |

Key message

Dietary restriction of calcium in stone formers is contraindicated.

Why it's important

The most common metabolic abnormality that is identified in patients with renal stones is idiopathic hypercalciuria. This may be found in 50% of stone formers. In this group, and also in patients with proven calcium oxalate stones but who are metabolically normal, the usual advice given, in an effort to reduce the potential for stone recurrence, was that patients should increase their fluid intake and reduce the amount of calcium in their diet. In this study, it was clearly shown that patients who consume more rather than less calcium have a lower incidence of stone recurrence. The possible mechanisms by which this might come about are discussed in the paper. The likelihood is that reduced calcium intake allows increased oxalate absorption. Furthermore, urinary oxalate may be more relevant than urinary calcium in terms of stone formation, because small increases in oxalate concentration in the urine have a disproportionately large effect on calcium oxalate saturation in the urine. The data from this paper would justify changing the metabolic advice that had for generations been given to patients with calcium oxalate stones.

Strengths

1. This was a large prospective study and was the first to investigate the association between dietary calcium restriction and recurrent stone formation.
2. Most previous studies have just looked at dietary calcium restriction in terms of the level of urinary calcium.

Weaknesses

1. In the questionnaire that was sent to patients, the oxalate values of different foods were assessed incompletely. The authors could not therefore show what could be thought of as a logical extrapolation of their findings, namely that increased oxalate ingestion would result in increased stone formation.
2. The questionnaire enquired only about food stuffs with high oxalate concentration (chocolate, nuts, tea and spinach), and the ingestion of these was not shown to be associated with an increased risk of stone relevance.

Relevance

There is often much debate about the need to study patients with renal stones metabolically. Some people believe that only recurrent stone formers should be offered a full metabolic screen, whereas others advocate that all patients who present with stones should be offered this investigation. The findings of this study could be regarded as support for screening all first-time stone formers. The relative lack of valid metabolic information on which to base advice is one of the principal findings of this paper. The authors provide data that reverse the usual advice given.

CHAPTER 15

Female urology

JOACHIM W THÜROFF, MD

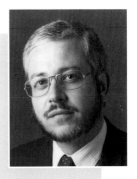

- 1976–1981: Resident in Pathology, Surgery and Urology in Marburg, Würzburg and Mainz, Germany
- 1981–1985: Assistant Professor, Dept. of Urology, Johannes Gutenburg University Medical School, Mainz, Germany
- 1985–1987: Associate Professor, Dept. of Urology, and Director, Urinary Stone Center, University of California Medical School, San Francisco, U.S.A.
- 1987–1997: Professor and Chairman, Dept. of Urology, Klinikum Barmen, University of Witten/Herdecke Medical School, Wuppertal, Germany
- Since 1997: Professor and Chairman, Dept. of Urology, Johannes Gutenberg University Medical School, Mainz, Germany

RUDOLF HOHENFELLNER, MD

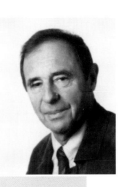

- 1953-1958: Resident in Surgery and Urology, University of Vienna Medical School, Vienna, Austria
- 1958–1964: Assistant Professor, Dept. of Urology, University of Vienna Medical School, Vienna, Austria
- 1964–1967: Associate Professor, Dept. of Urology, University of Saarland Medical School, Homburg/Saar, Germany
- 1967–1997: Professor and Chairman, Dept. of Urology, Johannes Gutenberg University Medical School, Mainz, Germany

MARCUS HOHENFELLNER, MD

Introduction

There are obvious dilemmas to select from numerous, mostly surgical papers on female incontinence that could be 'classics'. Those from Simms, Goebell, Aldrige, Burch and Martius are early (first?) descriptions of techniques, the original techniques or surgical principles that have, over time, proved to be useful and thus have survived with or without major modifications. The paper by Marchetti has reported an important modification of the original technique by Marshall, Marchetti and Krantz. That by Stanton was the first to perform a comparative trial between anterior vaginal repair and retropubic colposuspension. That by Kegel has founded the principles of pelvic floor exercises controlled by biofeedback and Enhörning gave a detailed and precise description of physiology and pathophysiology of the urethral sphincteric mechanisms as described by urethral pressure measurement. Finally, Bates *et al.* founded the International Continence Society's standardization of terminology and assessment of lower urinary tract function and produced a classification of urinary incontinence.

Title

Zur operativen Beseitigung der angeborenen incontinentia vesicae [The operative cure for congenital incontinentia vesicae]

Author

Goebell R

Reference

Zeitschrift für gynäkologische Urologie 1910; **2**: 187–191

Abstract

Not available

Summary

Social continence was achieved using the pyramidal muscle for bladder neck reconstruction in two incontinent patients with the underlying conditions of myelomeningocele and bladder exstrophy. The muscle was wrapped around the bladder neck and the ends rejoined.

Citation count	43

Related reference (1)	Ridley JH. The Goebell–Stoeckel sling operation. In: *TeLinde's Operative Gynecology* (Mattingly RF, Thompson JD, eds), 4th edn. Philadelphia: JB Lippincott, 1985: 923–935.
Related reference (2)	Jarvis GJ. Surgery for genuine stress incontinence: Review. *British Journal of Obstetrics and Gynaecology* 1994; **101**: 371–374.
Related reference (3)	Wall LL, Copas P, Galloway NTM. Use of the pedicled rectus abdominis muscle flap sling in the treatment of complicated stress incontinence. *American Journal of Obstetrics and Gynecology* 1996; **175**: 140–146.

Key message

This paper provided the first description of a successful, muscle-sling, bladder-neck plasty in patients with exstrophy and myelomeningocele. It was the prototype from which all following fascial and muscular sling plasties in the twentieth century were copied and developed.

Why it's important

Instead of purse-string sutures placed around the bladder neck, for the first time a muscular ring plasty was employed for the treatment of urinary incontinence. Emphasis is put on avoiding injury to the bladder or vagina by careful dissection of the vesicovaginal septum, which is described in detail. The author provided the blueprint for all ensuing urethral and anal sphincter ring and sling plasties.

Strengths

1. Simple and reproducible concept and technique.
2. Detailed description to avoid complications.
3. Describes the dissection of the vesiocovaginal septum.
4. Discusses the use of alternative muscular structures, e.g. the gracilis muscle.

Weaknesses

1. The concept of voluntary muscular contraction for bladder closure was wrong.
2. Two cases only, with insufficient follow-up.

Relevance

All later bladder neck reconstructions in bladder exstrophy follow this basic principle. It allows for controlled bladder-neck obstruction.

Title

Transplantation of fascia for relief of urinary stress incontinence

Author

Aldridge AH

Reference

American Journal of Obstetrics and Gynecology 1942; 398–411

Abstract

Not available

Summary

Detailed description (ten figures, 'step-by-step') of an incontinence procedure, which was referred to as the 'Aldrige sling' in the subsequent literature. The combined suprapubic and transvaginal approach was based on the surgical concept developed by Goebell almost 30 years earlier. The technique was successfully applied in a 53-year-old woman with severe day- and night-time incontinence after the failure of several other surgical interventions.

Citation count	59
Related reference (1)	McGuire EJ, Lytton B. The pubovaginal sling for stress urinary incontinence. *Journal of Urology* 1978; **119**: 82.
Related reference (2)	Eckford SD, Bailey RA, Jackson SR, Shepherd AM, Abrams P. Occult pre-operative detrusor instability: an adverse prognostic feature in genuine stress incontinence surgery. *Neurourology and Urodynamics* 1995; **14**: 487–488.
Related reference (3)	Schumaker SA, Wyman SF, Uebersax JS. Health related quality of life measures for women with urinary incontinence: the Incontinence Impact Questionnaire and the Urogenital Distress Inventory. *Quality Life Research* 1994; **3**: 291–306.

Key message

This incontinence operation has stood the test of time and remains the gold standard. It can still be found in contemporary gynaecological textbooks without significant alterations.

Why it's important

A classic instructional piece for the, until then, unsolved problem of congenital urinary incontinence, and persisting urinary incontinence after multiple failed procedures. In spite of incomplete understanding of the urethral pathophysiology and with no experimental data from animal studies, an operative concept was derived from anatomical investigations and reports published in the German literature more than 30 years earlier. The case report impressively emphasizes the miserable quality of life with urinary incontinence and illustrates the often technically difficult situation after previous surgery.

Strengths

1. Admirable brainstorming led to the conclusive development of a standard procedure.
2. Impressive and clear presentation with excellent illustrations.
3. High reproducibility, low complication rate and good long-term results.

Weaknesses

1. Based on a single case.
2. No statistical data.

Relevance

The fascial sling has survived all artificial competitors and is irreplaceable in women with hypotonic urethra. This paper is an excellent example of the fact that it is always worth while to have a close look at the older surgical literature.

Title

Urinary incontinence

Author

Marchetti AA

Reference

Journal of the American Medical Association 1956; **162**: 1366–1368

Abstract

Not available

Summary

A modification of the Marshall–Marchetti–Krantz procedure (see Related reference (1)) is described, which was applied to 132 patients with stress urinary incontinence. One hundred and twenty-eight were followed for up to more than 10 years with a 84% cure rate.

Citation count	8

Related reference (1)   Marshall VF, Marchetti AA, Krantz KE. The correction of stress incontinence by simple vesicourethral suspension. *Surgery, Gynecology and Obstetrics* 1949; **88**: 509–518.

Related reference (2)   Burch JC. Urethrovaginal fixation to Cooper's ligament for correction of stress incontinence, cystocele, and prolapse. *American Journal of Obstetrics and Gynecology* 1961; **81**: 281–290.

Related reference (3)   McGuire EJ. Urodynamic findings in patients after failure of stress incontinence operations. In: *Female Incontinence* (Zinner NR, Sterling AM, eds). New York: Alan R. Liss, 1981: 351–360.

Key message

Retropubic suspension is an effective procedure to treat stress urinary incontinence. Suspension sutures should, however, not include the lateral wall of the urethra, as described in Related reference (1).

Why it's important

The original Marshall–Marchetti–Krantz procedure (see Related reference (1)) relied on suspension sutures that included the lateral wall of the urethra. This technique had two disadvantages: first, possible urethral damage and/or obstruction; second, inability to correct urethrocystoceles. The described modification of using colposuspension sutures instead of urethrocolposuspension sutures aimed at overcoming these disadvantages.

Strengths

1. Clear description of how stress incontinence should be diagnosed and how patients, who have mixed urge and stress incontinence, should be dealt with.
2. Detailed depiction of the surgical technique.
3. Special attention is given to placement of suspension sutures: exclusion of the urethral wall did avoid urethral damage and obstruction in this series. However, fixation to the periosteum of the pubis and the cartilage of the symphysis resulted in periostitis pubis in four cases.
4. Large patient collective and long-term follow-up with only a few drop-outs.

Weakness

1. Only rudimentary presentation of data.

Relevance

This paper is the basis for all following colposuspension procedures, such as the Burch colposuspension, which successfully solved Marchetti's problem with periostitis pubis.

Title

Urethrovaginal fixation to Cooper's ligament for correction of stress incontinence, cystocele, and prolapse

Author

Burch JC

Reference

American Journal of Obstetrics and Gynecology 1961; **81**: 281–290

Abstract

Not available

Summary

Between 1958 and 1960 the anterior vaginal wall was fixed to the Cooper's ligament ($n = 46$) and the white line ($n = 7$) in 53 patients. Their age ranged from 20 to 79 years with 35 women aged between 30 and 49 years. Hysterectomy ($n = 36$), posterior colporrhaphy and perineorrhaphy ($n = 45$) were performed in the same session. The complication rate was low (one vesicovaginal fistula, one ventral hernia, and recurrence of rectocele and enterocele in four). There were no failures in the 45 cases of stress urinary incontinence.

Citation count	234
Related reference (1)	Stanton SL, Cardozo LD. Results of colposuspension operation for incontinence and prolapse. *British Journal of Obstetrics and Gynaecology* 1979; **86**: 693.
Related reference (2)	Lose G, Jorgenson L, Mortenson SO, Molsted-Pedersen L, Kristensen JK. Voiding difficulties after colposuspension. *Obstetrics and Gynecology* 1978; **69**: 33–37.
Related reference (3)	Bown LW, Sand PK, Ostergard DR, Franti CE. Unsuccessful Burch retropubic urethropexy: a case-controlled urodynamic study. *American Journal of Obstetrics and Gynecology* 1989; **160**: 452–458.

Key message

This paper provided the first description of fixation of the anterior vaginal wall to Cooper's ligament, for curing female stress incontinence with a high success and a low complication rate. During the following 40 years, the 'Burch' procedure proved to be a gold standard, along with the Aldrige sling.

Why it's important

In contrast to the Marshall–Marchetti–Krantz procedure, Cooper's ligament provides an anatomically correct and stable 'anchor' for fixation of the anterior vaginal wall. The operation is easy to perform (controlled by one or two fingers pushing the anterior wall up), reproducible, and has a short learning curve with a low rate of early complications. Overcorrection is rare and the long-term results are favourable.

Strengths

1. Clear and simple message.
2. An example of an innovative idea born while addressing a similar question.
3. One of two techniques for stress urinary incontinence in women.

Weaknesses

1. The tissue of the anterior vaginal wall is of poor quality in elderly women.
2. Recurrence of stress incontinence after 5 years in up to 30% of all patients.

Relevance

This has replaced the Marshall–Marchetti–Krantz procedure.

Title

Comparison of anterior vaginal repair and retropubic colposuspension in the treatment of genuine stress incontinence

Author

Stanton SL

Reference

In: *Gynecologic Urology and Urodynamics* (Ostergard DR, ed.), 1st edn. Baltimore: Williams & Wilkins, 1980: 301–304

Abstract

Not available

Summary

Fifty unselected patients with urodynamically proven stress incontinence were subjected to one of two different surgical techniques for treatment of stress incontinence in a comparative trial. Twenty-five patients had an anterior vaginal repair and 25 a modified Burch colposuspension. The 6 months post-operative urodynamic evaluation revealed a 84% cure rate of the modified Burch colposuspension versus a 36% cure rate of anterior vaginal repair.

Citation count	2
Related reference (1)	Kelly HA. Incontinence of urine in women. *Urology and Cutaneous Review* 1913; **17**: 291.
Related reference (2)	Burch JC. Urethrovaginal fixation to Cooper's ligament for correction of stress incontinence, cystocele, and prolapse. *American Journal of Obstetrics and Gynecology* 1961; **81**: 281–290.
Related reference (3)	Alcalay M, Monga AK, Stanton SL. Burch colposuspension - how long does it cure stress incontinence? *Neurourology and Urodynamics* 1994; **13**: 495–497.

Key message

For the surgical treatment of stress incontinence, retropubic Burch colposuspension is effective, whereas anterior vaginal repair has an unacceptably low success rate.

Why it's important

Until this work was published, anterior vaginal repair had been performed in most cases for surgical treatment of stress urinary incontinence, especially by gynaecologists. Stanton's chapter describes the first comparative clinical trial evaluating the success of two surgical techniques in this field. It clearly demonstrated the superiority of retropubic colposuspension and the limited usefulness of anterior vaginal repair in the surgical treatment of stress urinary incontinence.

Strengths

1. Clinical comparative trial to assess the efficacy of two surgical procedures for treatment of stress incontinence.
2. Pre-operative and 6-month post-operative urodynamic corroboration of symptoms.

Weaknesses

1. Very general data presentation.
2. No statistics.
3. No pre-operative differentiation of the degree of stress incontinence.
4. No detailed presentation of urodynamic data.

Relevance

This work introduced comparative clinical trials for evaluation of surgical techniques in the treatment of stress incontinence, and promoted retropubic colposuspension for the treatment of stress incontinence. Anterior vaginal repair was no longer regarded as an adequate surgical procedure to cure stress incontinence.

Title

Die operative Wiederherstellung der vollkommen fehlenden Harnröhre und des Schließmuskels derselben [Surgical restoration of the completely absent urethra and its sphincteric muscle]

Author

Martius H

Reference

Zentralblatt für Gynäkologie 1928; **8**: 480–486

Abstract

Not available

Summary

Two major innovations are presented in one paper: (1) comprehensive description of a new technique for the reconstruction of the urethra involving the use of vaginal wall and ischiocavernosus muscle flaps, in a woman who had been incontinent for 5 years, despite three earlier attempts at reconstruction. The operation resulted in social continence (2–3 hours during the day, 6 hours at night). (2) Inauguration of the Martius labial fat-pad graft for reinforcement of suture lines in reconstructive procedures.

Citation count	35
Related reference (1)	Leach GE. Urethrovaginal fistula repair with Martius labial fat pad graft. *Urologic Clinics of North America* 1991; **18**: 409–413.
Related reference (2)	Hendren WH. Construction of female urethra from vaginal wall and a perineal flap. *Journal of Urology* 1980; **123**: 657–664.
Related reference (3)	Wein AJ, Malloy TR, Greenberg SH, Carpiniello VL, Murphy JJ. Omental transposition as an aid in genitourinary reconstructive procedures. *Journal of Trauma* 1980; **20**: 473–477.

Key message

The female urethra can be completely restored using a vaginal wall flap and flaps created from mobilized and pedicled bulbocavernosus and ischiocavernosus muscles. Whenever there is concern about the quality of vaginal tissues or the integrity of the reconstruction, a Martius labial fat-pad graft can be interposed to reinforce and cover the suture line.

Why it's important

Although Martius' name is more often associated with the labial fat-pad graft as the fore-runner of all later kinds of tissue interposition (omentum, gracilis muscle, peritoneum) in reconstructive surgery, he was also the pioneer in using pedicled flaps in the restoration of the urethra. The latest variations on the same theme are the full-thickness bladder wall flap in continent vesicostomy and the bowel flaps used for the creation of continence mechanisms in urinary diversion.

Strengths

1. Two important concepts in one paper.
2. Applicable in salvage manoeuvres after previously failed reconstruction.
3. The muscular tissue of the neourethra originates from an untouched, 'healthy' area.

Weaknesses

1. Based on a single case.
2. Continence achieved through unpredictable degree of obstruction.
3. No voluntary muscular bladder closure.

Relevance

The technique described allows restoration of social continence in otherwise hopeless cases. The approach has the obvious advantage of avoiding a major transabdominal procedure. The interposition of healthy tissue to protect suture lines is a must in reconstructive urology. Both ideas found widespread application in various modifications.

Title

On the treatment of vesico-vaginal fistula

Authors

Simms JM

Reference

American Journal of the Medical Sciences 1852; **23**: 59

Abstract

Not available

Summary

The author provides a conclusive classification of fistulae based on their location. A step-by-step description of a new method is given, including details on the patient's position (knee elbow), a new suture apparatus, a self-retaining catheter and post-operative care. The basic principle of the technique involves: (1) a funnel-shaped circumcision of the fistula to create a shallow crater; (2) minimal mobilization of the vaginal mucosa; and (3) everting sutures through the vaginal epithelium and the detrusor muscle.

Citation count	Not available
Related reference (1)	Jonas U, Petri E. Genitourinary fistulae. In: *Clinical Gynaecologic Urology* (Stanton SL, ed.). St Louis, CV Mosby Co., 1984: 238–255.
Related reference (2)	Goodwin WE, Scardino PT. Vesicovaginal and ureterovaginal fistulas: a summary of 25 years of experience. *Journal of Urology* 1980; **123**: 370–374.
Related reference (3)	Blaivas JG, Heritz DM, Romanzi LJ. Early versus late repair of vesico-vaginal fistulas: vaginal and abdominal approaches. *Journal of Urology* 1995; **153**: 1110–1113.

Key message

This paper is the first description of a simple and reproducible method to cure fistulae between the bladder and the vagina by a transvaginal approach. It achieved high popularity with numerous modifications.

Why it's important

All previous procedures used for fistula closure proved to be insufficient. It is demonstrated that patient positioning, and especially developed instruments (source of light incorporated in a speculum) and the choice of suture material are important factors that contribute to a successful realization of a logical concept.

Strengths

1. Comprehensive description of all relevant operative steps; it is reproducible.
2. Provides a practicable answer to a hitherto unsolved surgical problem.
3. Less damaging approach (vaginal access).
4. Minimal mobilization, avoidance of dead space and minimal suture material.

Weaknesses

1. A detailed description of the complications is lacking.
2. No statistical analysis was carried out.

Relevance

Before the efforts of dedicated surgeons such as James Marion Simms, urinary fistulae were generally considered to be intractable, with the affected woman doomed to a life in social isolation. Through his innovations in surgical technique and the routine use of post-operative drainage of the bladder using a self-retaining catheter, for the first time Simms offered a reasonable chance for cure. More than 100 years later, and popularized by Moir, it remains a standard vaginal procedure.

Title

Physiologic treatment of poor tone and function of the genital muscles and of urinary stress incontinence

Author

Kegel AH

Reference

Western Journal of Surgery 1949; **57**: 527–535

Abstract

Not available

Summary

The pathophysiology of pelvic floor dysfunction in relation to urinary stress incontinence is described. Diagnosis of poor tone and function of the pelvic floor muscles by physical examination and the use of a vaginal pressure manometer, and their treatment by physical exercise are introduced. Several clinical presentations are given: (1) urinary stress incontinence; (2) post-menopausal atrophy of the perivaginal muscle; (3) persistent postpartum relaxation of the genital muscles; and (4) poor tone and function of the genital muscles during the child-bearing years.

Citation count	25

Related reference (1) Bo K. Adherence to pelvic floor muscle exercise and long-term effect on stress urinary incontinence. A 5-year follow-up study. *Scandinavian Journal of Medical Science and Sports* 1995; **5**: 36–39.

Related reference (2) Peattie AB, Plevnik S. Cones versus physiotherapy as conservative management of genuine stress incontinence. *Neurourology and Urodynamics* 1988; **7**: 265–266.

Related reference (3) Berghmans LC, Hendriks HJ, Bo K, Hay-Smith EJ, de Bie RA, van Waalwijk van Doorn ES. Conservative treatment of stress urinary incontinence in women: a systematic review of randomized clinical trials. *British Journal of Urology* 1998; **82**: 181–191.

Key message

Stress incontinence may be a result of poor tone and function of the pelvic floor muscles. These can be corrected by active exercise using biofeedback techniques for re-education in the control of function and coordination of the neuromuscular structures of the pelvic floor.

Why it's important

This paper has founded a new theory of diagnosis and treatment of neuromuscular pelvic floor dysfunction, based on the concept of atrophy of striated muscles through disuse. It introduced biofeedback principles (contraction pressure re-evaluation) as a valuable tool to the therapeutic arsenal of pelvic floor exercises in the treatment of urinary stress incontinence; up to this point only surgical solutions had been employed.

Strengths

1. Excellent description of the pathophysiology of neuromuscular pelvic floor dysfunction, based on phylogenetic, anatomical and physiological objectives.
2. The diagnostic interventions, as well as the use of biofeedback for pelvic floor exercises, have remained as the standard until today.
3. The clinical case reports are 'to the point'.

Weaknesses

1. No stratification of patient collectives with neuromuscular pelvic floor dysfunction in which biofeedback may and may not work (e.g. with gross denervation of pelvic floor muscles).
2. No mention of failures and possible explanations.
3. No cumulative data on patients, therapeutic regimens and follow-up.

Relevance

This paper provided the first description of biofeedback for exercising the pelvic floor muscles.

Title

Simultaneous recording of intravesical and intra-urethral pressure

Author

Enhörning G

Reference

Acta Chirurgica Scandinavia 1961; **276**(suppl): 1–68

Abstract

Not available

Summary

Two hundred and six women were subjected to simultaneous pressure measurements in the bladder and urethra; 111 were classified as normal, 65 as stress incontinent and 30 as puerperant.

Citation count	194

Related reference (1)	Graber P, Laurent G, Tanagho EA. Effect of abdominal pressure rise on the urethral profile. *Investigative Urology* 1974; **12**: 57–64.
Related reference (2)	Heidler H, Wölk H, Jonas U. Urethral closure under stress conditions. *European Urology* 1979; **5**: 110–112.
Related reference (3)	Thüroff JW, Bazeed MA, Schmidt RA, Tanagho EA. Mechanisms of urinary continence: an animal model to study urethral responses to stress conditions. *Journal of Urology* 1982; **127**: 1202.

Key message

Continence under stress conditions, such as coughing, is physiologically warranted by transmission of abdominal pressure to the part of the urethra that is located above the pelvic floor, and by contraction of striated urethral sphincter and pelvic floor muscles at the level of the mid-urethra. Women with stress incontinence may be treated by surgical procedures that allow (re)exposure of the urethra to intra-abdominal forces.

Why it's important

This is the first paper to describe simultaneous independent pressure measurements in the human urethra and the bladder under physiological conditions. It explores and proves the presence and mechanism of abdominal-urethral pressure transmission, and reflex or voluntary contraction of striated sphincteric muscles.

Strengths

1. Clear hypothesis.
2. Meticulous methodology, including development, calibration, and application of catheters and pressure transducers.
3. Control group.
4. Statistical analysis.

Weakness

1. It recognizes only reduced abdominal-urethral pressure transmission and defective reflex contraction of striated sphincteric muscles as causes of incontinence; it does not recognize other pathological entities, for example, hypotonic urethra (intrinsic sphincter deficiency; type III incontinence) and deficiencies of the epithelial closure pressure.

Relevance

This paper is the basis for understanding the pathophysiology of stress urinary incontinence. It stimulated contemporary diagnostic urodynamic approaches and treatment strategies.

Title

First report on the standardization of terminology of lower urinary tract function

Authors

Bates P, Bradley WE, Glen E, Melchior H, Rowan D, Sterling A, Hald T

References

British Journal of Urology 1976; **48**: 39–42
European Urology 1976; **2**: 274–276
Scandinavian Journal of Urology and Nephrology 1977; **11**: 193–196
Urologia Internationalis (Basel) 1977; **32**: 81–87

Abstract

Not available

Summary

This paper provided the first proposal of recommendations for standardization of the terminology of lower urinary tract function and dysfunction. The report was the result of a business meeting of the International Continence Society (ICS) in 1974, which focused on the storage function of the bladder, classification of urinary incontinence, cystometry, urethral closure pressure profile and units of measurement.

Citation count	38 (total)
Related reference (1)	Abrams P, Blaivas JG, Stanton SL, Andersen JT. The standardization of the lower urinary tract function. The International Continence Society. *Scandinavian Journal of Urology and Nephrology* 1988; **114**(suppl): 5–19.
Related reference (2)	Andersen JT, Blaivas JG, Cardozo L, Thüroff JW. Seventh report on standardization of lower urinary tract function. Lower urinary tract rehabilitation techniques. The International Continence Society. *Scandinavian Journal of Urology and Nephrology* 1992; **26**: 99–106.
Related reference (3)	Thüroff JW, Mattiasson A, Andersen JT, Hedlund H, Hinman F Jr, Hohenfellner M *et al.* The standardization of terminology and assessment of functional characteristics of intestinal urinary reservoirs. International Continence Society, Committee on Standardization of Terminology. Subcommittee on Intestinal Urinary Reservoirs. *British Journal of Urology* 1996; **78**: 516–523.

Key message

This paper gave a description of lower urinary tract function and dysfunction in standardized and generally accepted terms and definitions, allowing international comparison of trials in this field. The terms and their definitions, which are outlined in this report, are the consensus of the ICS, an interdisciplinary scientific association of urologists, gynaecologists, specialist nurses and engineers.

Why it's important

This paper instigated the initiation of a worldwide consensus effort to use standardized terminology for lower urinary tract function and dysfunction and - where possible - standardized techniques and documentation of results in urodynamic assessments.

Strengths

1. Very concise paper explaining urodynamic key points in a comprehensive and broadly understandable way.
2. Classification of urinary incontinence.
3. Exact definition of terms of dysfunction.
4. Recommendations of which units of measurement should be used.

Weaknesses

1. Over-emphasizes urinary storage dysfunction.
2. Neglects voiding dysfunctions (e.g. detrusor–sphincter dys-synergia).
3. No consensus in the recommendation of standardized techniques of urodynamic assessment (it was agreed, however, always to record exactly how the urodynamic evaluation was performed [e.g. liquid or gas cystometry in a supine, sitting or standing position]).

Relevance

This paper was a first step in the standardization of urodynamic terms and definitions. It provided a basic framework for all subsequent standardization reports. It was a prerequisite for current diagnostic and therapeutic procedures in the evaluation of lower urinary tract function. Without such efforts, development of computer-assisted urodynamic diagnostic equipment, and conduction of multicentre trials of therapeutic interventions such as pharmacotherapy, would have been very difficult.

The Top 100 Papers in Urology

This is the first time that an attempt has been made to list the one hundred most quoted papers in urology; but before we get inundated with letters from authors who feel they have been overlooked, or are heavily criticised by semi-professional scrutinisers of citation indices (we know you exist), let us explain how we compiled this list.

The first problem is that from a publication point of view there is no such thing as urology. Enter the term 'urology' into any search engine and you will get far fewer hits than you might think. 'Urology' is not often used as a key word, nor is it indexed as part of the Medical Subject Headings (MESH) on electronic databases such as Medline. An alternative approach might be to use urological organs as a basis for a search strategy: at least any article with the words 'prostate' or 'testicle' would be identified. The trouble with this approach is immediately obvious. A search using the words 'renal' or 'kidney' would generate plenty of articles but by far the majority would be non-urological, however you chose to define the term. Articles on hypertension alone would greatly outnumber the combined articles that most of us would consider urological.

Our approach was as follows. Our list would comprise two distinct searches. One set of papers would come from a search designed to establish the most cited papers in journals that most of us would call urological. This is a long but certainly not exhaustive list: last year alone we were aware of at least three new journals dedicated to diseases of the prostate. The strength of this type of approach is that editors are unlikely to publish articles that are not of interest to the urologist; the trouble with this approach is that the search is time sensitive. If one does not restrict the search to a defined period, say the last ten years, then articles that appeared long ago and therefore have been quoted over the years will tend be at the top of the list. A search confined to the period 1981 to 1997 (Table 1) of the titles listed below gave Oesterling's paper on PSA (*J Urol* 1991; 145: 907) the top position with 538 citations. The same search from a different database, this time confined to the years 1935 to 1992 (Table 2), listed Robson's paper on the results of radical nephrectomy (*J Urol* 1969; 101: 297) as the most cited paper, with 498 citations.

This, however, was not the main bias associated with this strategy. When authors feel they have something important to say they prefer to shout the message to the whole medical community rather than whisper it to their urological colleagues. This is particularly true for disciplines such as molecular biology. Authors will submit the better articles to specialist journals read by scientists undertaking similar types of work. Again, if it is difficult to compile a list of urological journals then it is nearly impossible to compile a list of general and specialist journals where papers of urological interest are likely to appear.

To overcome this we relied on our expert selectors. Every paper that was deemed to be worthy of inclusion in *Classic Papers in Urology* was put in a search to determine how many times it had been cited (Table 3). You will see that the top three spots are all occupied by classic papers that were published in general rather than urological journals (*Ann Int Med*, *Can Res* and *N Engl J Med*), one as long ago as 1941.

Thus the list in Table 3 is as close as we can get to one that includes the papers that urological authors consider important enough to quote on a frequent basis. There are a few surprises and some interesting trends. We hope that this league table will, as all league tables tend to do, stimulate both thought and debate on the papers our expert selectors have chosen to include or leave out of their list of classic papers in urology.

Mark Emberton

Acknowledgement

Data for Tables 1, 2 and 3, and all citation counts appearing in this book, was provided by the Institute for Scientific Information (ISI) (*http: //www.isinet.com*). Our thanks to ISI for their help in this matter.

Appendix: Journals searched for data in Tables

- Akt Urol
- Ann Urol
- Br J Urol
- Eur Urol
- Infect Urol
- J Endourol
- J Urol
- J Urologie
- Mol Urol
- Neurourol U
- Prostate
- Prostate C
- Scand J Urol Nephrol
- Urol Clin N Am
- Urol Intern
- Urol Res
- Urologe
- Urology
- Urol Surv
- World J Urol

Table 1: The 100 most cited papers in urology, 1981–1997 *

Bold text = paper appears in *Classic Papers in Urology*

Position	Citation count	Author	Paper title	Journal, date, volume, page no.
1	538	Oesterling JE	Prostate specific antigen – a critical assessment of the most useful tumor marker for adenocarcinoma of the prostate	J Urol 1991, 145, 907
2	465	**Mebust WK**	**Transurethral prostatectomy: immediate and post-operative complications. A cooperative study of 13 participating institutions evaluating 3,885 patients**	**J Urol 1989, 141, 243–247**
3	388	**Berry SJ**	**The development of human benign prostatic hyperplasia with age**	**J Urol 1984, 132, 474–479**
4	384	Stamey TA	Prostate specific antigen in the diagnosis and treatment of adenocarcinoma of the prostate. 2. radical prostatectomy treated patients	J Urol 1989, 141, 1076
5	370	Oesterling JE	Prostate specific antigen in the pre-operative and post-operative evaluation of localized prostatic cancer treated with radical prostatectomy	J Urol 1988, 139, 766
6	342	Cooner WH	Prostate cancer detection in a clinical urological practice by ultrasonography, digital rectal examination and prostate specific antigen	J Urol 1990, 143, 1146
7	324	Drach GW	Report of the United States cooperative study of extracorporeal shock-wave lithotripsy	J Urol 1986, 135, 1127
8	320	Lange PH	The value of serum prostate specific antigen determinations before and after radical prostatectomy	J Urol 1989, 141, 873
9	315	**Barry MJ**	**The American Urological Association symptom index for benign prostatic hyperplasia**	**J Urol 1992, 148, 1,549–1,557**
10	315	Hudson MA	Clinical use of prostate specific antigen in patients with prostate cancer	J Urol 1989, 142, 1011
11	314	Chaussy C	1st clinical experience with extracorporeally induced destruction of kidney stones by shock-waves	J Urol 1982, 127, 417
12	307	Lue TF	Physiology of erection and pharmacological management of impotence	J Urol 1987, 137, 829

13	Heney NM	Superficial bladder cancer – progression and recurrence	J Urol 1983, 130, 1083–1086
14	Walsh PC	Impotence following radical prostatectomy – insight into etiology and prevention	J Urol 1982, 128, 492
15	Kock NG	Urinary diversion via a continent ileal reservoir – clinical results in 12 patients	J Urol 1982, 128, 469–475
16	Catalona WJ	Comparison of digital rectal examination and serum prostate-specific antigen in the early detection of prostate cancer – results of a multicenter clinical trial of 6,630 men	J Urol 1994, 151, 1283
17	Partin AW	Prostate specific antigen in the staging of localized prostate cancer – influence of tumor differentiation, tumor volume and benign hyperplasia	J Urol 1990, 143, 747
18	Partin AW	The use of prostate-specific antigen, clinical stage and Gleason score to predict pathological stage in men with localized prostate cancer	J Urol 1993, 150, 110
19	Brawer MK	Screening for prostatic carcinoma with prostate specific antigen	J Urol 1992, 147, 841
20	Zorgniotti AW	Auto-injection of the corpus cavernosum with a vasoactive drug-combination for vasculogenic impotence	J Urol 1985, 133, 39
21	Christensson A	Serum prostate-specific antigen complexed to alpha-1–antichymotrypsin as an indicator of prostate cancer	J Urol 1993, 150, 100
22	Benson MC	The use of prostate specific antigen density to enhance the predictive value of intermediate levels of serum prostate specific antigen	J Urol 1992, 147, 817
23	McGuire EJ	Prognostic value of urodynamic testing in myelodysplastic patients	J Urol 1981, 126, 205–209
24	Walsh PC	Radical prostatectomy with preservation of sexual function – anatomical and pathological considerations	Prostate 1983, 4, 473–485
25	Stamey TA	Morphometric and clinical studies on 68 consecutive radical prostatectomies	J Urol 1988, 139, 1235
26	Benson MC	Prostate specific antigen density – a means of distinguishing benign prostatic hypertrophy and prostate cancer	J Urol 1992, 147, 815
27	Sternberg CN	Preliminary results of M-VAC (methotrexate, vinblastine, doxorubicin and cisplatin) for transitional cell carcinoma of the urothelium	J Urol 1985, 133, 403

28	Partin AW	Serum PSA after anatomic radical prostatectomy – the Johns Hopkins experience after 10 years	Urol Clin N Am 1993, 20, 713
29	**Sternberg CN**	**M-VAC (methotrexate, vinblastine, doxorubicin and cisplatin) for advanced transitional cell carcinoma of the urothelium**	**J Urol 1988, 139, 461–469**
30	Brosman SA	Experience with bacillus Calmette–Guérin in patients with superficial bladder carcinoma	J Urol 1982, 128, 27
31	Cantrell BB	Pathological factors that influence prognosis in stage A prostatic cancer: the influence of extent versus grade	J Urol 1981, 125, 516
32	Paulson DF	Radical surgery versus radiotherapy for adenocarcinoma of the prostate	J Urol 1982, 128, 502
33	Stamey TA	Prostate specific antigen in the diagnosis and treatment of adenocarcinoma of the prostate. 1. untreated patients	J Urol 1989, 141, 1070
34	Hodge KK	Random systematic versus directed ultrasound guided trans-rectal core biopsies of the prostate	J Urol 1989, 142, 71
35	Ercole CJ	Prostatic specific antigen and prostatic acid-phosphatase in the monitoring and staging of patients with prostatic cancer	J Urol 1987, 138, 1181
36	Schreiber MJ	The natural history of atherosclerotic and fibrous renal artery disease	Urol Clin N Am 1984, 11, 383
37	Labrie F	New approach in the treatment of prostate cancer – complete instead of partial withdrawal of androgens	Prostate 1983, 4, 579
38	Lutzeyer W	Prognostic parameters in superficial bladder cancer – an analysis of 315 cases	J Urol 1982, 127, 250
39	Bloom HJG	Treatment of T3 bladder cancer – controlled trial of pre-operative radiotherapy and radical cystectomy versus radical radiotherapy – 2nd report and review for the Clinical Trials Group, Institute Of Urology	Br J Urol 1982, 54, 136
40	Carter HB	The prostate – an increasing medical problem	Prostate 1990, 16, 39
41	Clayman RV	Laparoscopic nephrectomy – initial case report	J Urol 1991, 146, 278
42	Lingeman JE	Extracorporeal shock-wave lithotripsy – the Methodist Hospital of Indiana experience	J Urol 1986, 135, 1134
43	Tribukait B	The significance of ploidy and proliferation in the clinical and biological evaluation of bladder tumors – a study of 100 untreated cases	Br J Urol 1982, 54, 130

Ref	Author	Title	Page	Citation
44	Tribukait B	Flow cytometry in assessing the clinical aggressiveness of genitourinary neoplasms	183	World J Urol 1987, 5, 108
45	Isaacs JT	Establishment and characterization of 7 Dunning rat prostatic cancer cell lines and their use in developing methods for predicting metastatic abilities of prostatic cancers	181	Prostate 1986, 9, 261
46	McNichols DW	Renal cell carcinoma – long-term survival and late recurrence	178	J Urol 1981, 126, 17
47	Lue TF	Hemodynamics of erection in the monkey	175	J Urol 1983, 130, 1237
48	Lamm DL	Bacillus Calmette–Guérin immunotherapy for bladder cancer	173	J Urol 1985, 134, 40
49	Hedlund H	Effects of prazosin in patients with benign prostatic obstruction	172	J Urol 1983, 130, 275
50	Lamm DL	Complications of bacillus Calmette–Guérin immunotherapy in 1,278 patients with bladder cancer	171	J Urol 1986, 135, 272
51	Lieber MM	Renal oncocytoma	171	J Urol 1981, 125, 481
52	Fowler FJ	Patient-reported complications and follow-up treatment after radical prostatectomy – the national Medicare experience – 1988–1990. Updated June 1993	170	Urology 1993, 42, 622
53	Labrie F	Serum prostate specific antigen as pre-screening test for prostate cancer	170	J Urol 1992, 147, 846
54	Murphy GP	The national survey of prostate cancer in the United States by the American College of Surgeons	170	J Urol 1982, 127, 928
55	Epstein JI	Prognosis of untreated stage-AI prostatic carcinoma – a study of 94 cases with extended follow-up	169	J Urol 1986, 136, 837
56	Catalona WJ	Nerve-sparing radical prostatectomy – evaluation of results after 250 patients	167	J Urol 1990, 143, 538
57	Wang MC	Prostate antigen – a new potential marker for prostatic cancer	167	Prostate 1981, 2, 89
58	Chaussy C	Extracorporeal shock-wave lithotripsy (ESWL) for treatment of urolithiasis	166	Urology 1984, 23, 59
59	Diokno AC	Prevalence of urinary incontinence and other urological symptoms in the noninstitutionalized elderly	165	J Urol 1986, 136, 1022
60	Kabalin JN	Identification of residual cancer in the prostate following radiation therapy – role of trans-rectal ultrasound guided biopsy and prostate specific antigen	161	J Urol 1989, 142, 326

#		Author	Title	Reference
61	161	Schuessler WW	Transperitoneal endosurgical lymphadenectomy in patients with localized prostate cancer	J Urol 1991, 145, 988
62	160	Holtgrewe HL	Trans-urethral prostatectomy – practice aspects of the dominant operation in American urology	J Urol 1989, 141, 248
63	159	Kirby RS	Prazosin in the treatment of prostatic obstruction – a placebo-controlled study	Br J Urol 1987, 60, 136
64	158	Stamey TA	Prostate specific antigen in the diagnosis and treatment of adenocarcinoma of the prostate. 3. radiation treated patients	J Urol 1989, 141, 1084
65	156	Costello AJ	Laser ablation of the prostate in patients with benign prostatic hypertrophy	Br J Urol 1992, 69, 603
66	156	Rowland RG	Indiana continent urinary reservoir	J Urol 1987, 137, 1136
67	**155**	**Ball AJ**	**The natural history of untreated prostatism**	**Br J Urol 1981, 53, 613**
68	155	Lepor H	A randomized, placebo-controlled multicenter study of the efficacy and safety of terazosin in the treatment of benign prostatic hyperplasia	J Urol 1992, 148, 1467
69	155	Steinberg GD	Family history and the risk of prostate cancer	Prostate 1990, 17, 337
70	154	Paulson DF	Radical prostatectomy for clinical stage T1–2N0M0 prostatic adenocarcinoma – long-term results	J Urol 1990, 144, 1180
71	148	English HF	Relationship between DNA fragmentation and apoptosis in the programmed cell death in the rat prostate following castration	Prostate 1989, 15, 233
72	**147**	**Alken P**	**Percutaneous stone manipulation**	**J Urol 1981, 125, 463**
73	147	Caine M	The present role of alpha-adrenergic blockers in the treatment of benign prostatic hypertrophy	J Urol 1986, 136, 1
74	146	Lee F	Trans-rectal ultrasound in the diagnosis of prostate cancer – location, echogenicity, histopathology, and staging	Prostate 1985, 7, 117
75	146	Skinner DG	Clinical-experience with the Kock continent ileal reservoir for urinary diversion	J Urol 1984, 132, 1101
76	146	Stein A	Prostate specific antigen levels after radical prostatectomy in patients with organ confined and locally extensive prostate cancer	J Urol 1992, 147, 942
77	142	Feldman HA	Impotence and its medical and psychosocial correlates – results of the Massachusetts male aging study	J Urol 1994, 151, 54

78	Kabalin JN	Laser prostatectomy performed with a right-angle firing neodymium-YAG laser fiber at 40 watts power setting	J Urol 1993, 150, 95
79	Denis LJ	Goserelin acetate and flutamide versus bilateral orchiectomy – a phase-III EORTC trial (30853)	Urology 1993, 42, 119
80	Gervasi LA	Prognostic significance of lymph nodal metastases in prostate cancer	J Urol 1989, 142, 332
81	Stamey TA	Prostate specific antigen in the diagnosis and treatment of adenocarcinoma of the prostate. 4. anti-androgen treated patients	J Urol 1989, 141, 1088
82	Gibbons RP	Total prostatectomy for localized prostatic cancer	J Urol 1984, 131, 73
83	Montpetit ML	Androgen-repressed messages in the rat ventral prostate	Prostate 1986, 8, 25
84	Segura JW	Percutaneous removal of kidney stones – review of 1,000 cases	J Urol 1985, 134, 1077
85	Cooner WH	Clinical application of trans-rectal ultrasonography and prostate specific antigen in the search for prostate cancer	J Urol 1988, 139, 758
86	Lilien OM	25 year experience with replacement of the human bladder (Camey procedure)	J Urol 1984, 132, 886
87	Chute CG	The prevalence of prostatism – a population-based survey of urinary symptoms	J Urol 1993, 150, 85
88	Diamond DA	A new method to assess metastatic potential of human prostate cancer – relative nuclear roundness	J Urol 1982, 128, 729
89	Gustafson H	DNA profile and tumor progression in patients with superficial bladder tumors	Urol Res 1982, 10, 13
90	Lue TF	Functional evaluation of penile veins by cavernosography in papaverine-induced erection	J Urol 1986, 135, 479
91	Partin AW	The clinical usefulness of prostate-specific antigen – update 1994	J Urol 1994, 152, 1358
92	Raz S	Modified bladder neck suspension for female stress-incontinence	Urology 1981, 17, 82
93	Trachtenberg J	Correlation of prostatic nuclear androgen receptor content with duration of response and survival following hormonal therapy in advanced prostatic cancer	J Urol 1982, 127, 466
94	Freiha FS	Carcinoma of the prostate – results of post-irradiation biopsy	Prostate 1984, 5, 19
95	Katz AE	Molecular staging of prostate cancer with the use of an enhanced reverse-transcriptase PCR assay	Urology 1994, 43, 765

96	Abrams P	Standardization of terminology of lower urinary tract function	Neurourol U 1988, 7, 403
97	Elder JS	Radical perineal prostatectomy for clinical stage-B2 carcinoma of the prostate	J Urol 1982, 127, 704
98	Herr HW	An overview of intravesical therapy for superficial bladder tumors	J Urol 1987, 138, 1363
99	Herr HW	Long-term effect of intravesical bacillus Calmette–Guérin on flat carcinoma *in situ* of the bladder	J Urol 1986, 135, 265
100	Schmidt JD	Trends in patterns of care for prostatic cancer, 1974–1983 – results of surveys by the American College of Surgeons	J Urol 1986, 136, 416

* Citation counts provided by ISI.

Table 2: The 100 most cited papers in urology, 1935–1992 * †

Bold text = paper appears in *Classic Papers in Urology*

Position	Citation count	Author	Paper title	Journal, date, volume, page no.
1	498	Robson CJ	The results of radical nephrectomy for renal cell carcinoma	J Urol 1969, 101, 297
2	472	Gleason DF	Prediction of prognosis for prostatic adenocarcinoma by combined histological grading and clinical staging	J Urol 1974, 111, 58
3	404	**Politano VA**	**An operative technique for the correction of vesicoureteral reflux**	**J Urol 1958, 79, 932–941**
4	399	Jewett HJ	Infiltrating carcinoma of the bladder. Relation of depth of penetration of the bladder wall to incidence of local extension and metastases	J Urol 1946, 55, 366
5	382	Herbut P	†	In: Myron Tannebaum (Editor) Urological Pathology, Lea & Febiger, Philadelphia, 1977
6	370	**Gleason DF & the VACURG**	**Histologic grading and clinical staging of prostate carcinoma**	**In: Myron Tannebaum (Editor) Urological Pathology, Lea & Febiger, Philadelphia, 1977, 171–197**
7	347	Ormond JK	Bilateral ureteral obstruction due to envelopment and compression by an inflammatory retroperitoneal process	J Urol 1948, 59, 1072
8	334	Berger J	Les depot intercapillaries d'IgA–IgG	J Urologie 1968, 74, 694
9	325	Brown M	The urethral pressure profile	Brit J Urol 1969, 41, 211
10	317	**Morales A et al**	**Intracavitary bacillus Calmette–Guérin in the treatment of superficial bladder tumours**	**J Urol 1976, 116, 180–183**
11	308	Franzen S	Cytological diagnosis of prostatic tumours by transrectal aspiration biopsy: a preliminary report	Brit J Urol 1960, 32, 193
12	305	Oesterling J	Prostate specific antigen – a critical assessment of the most useful tumor marker for adenocarcinoma of the prostate	J Urol 1991, 145, 907
13	286	Stamey TA	Prostate specific antigen in the diagnosis and treatment of adenocarcinoma of the prostate. II. radical prostatectomy treated patients	J Urol 1989, 141, 1076

		Author	Title	Citation
14	285	Drach GW	Report of the United States cooperative study of extracorporeal shock-wave lithotripsy	J Urol 1986, 135, 1127
15	284	Jewett HJ	The present status of radical prostatectomy for stages A and B prostatic cancer	Urol Clin N Am Am 1975, 2, 105
16	283	Chaussy C	1st clinical experience with extracorporeally induced destruction of kidney stones by shock-waves	J Urol 1982, 127, 417
17	282	Prien EL	Studies in urolithiasis: I. The composition of urinary calculi	J Urol 1947, 57, 949
18	269	Oesterling J	Prostate specific antigen in the pre-operative and post-operative evaluation of localized prostatic cancer treated with radical prostatectomy	J Urol 1988, 139, 766
19	263	**Mebust WK**	**Trans-urethral prostatectomy – immediate and post-operative complications – a cooperative study of 13 participating institutions evaluating 3,885 patients**	**J Urol 1989, 141, 243**
20	262	**Lapides J et al**	**Clean intermittent self-catheterization in the treatment of urinary tract disease**	**J Urol 1972, 107, 458–461**
21	255	Mostofi FK	Potentialities of bladder epithelium	J Urol 1954, 71, 705
22	240	**Kock NG**	**Urinary diversion via a continent ileal reservoir: clinical results in 12 patients**	**J Urol 1982, 128, 469**
23	237	Cooner WH	Prostate cancer detection in a clinical urological practice by ultrasonography, digital rectal examination and prostate specific antigen	J Urol 1990, 143, 1146
24	236	Cox CE	Experiments with induced bacteriuria, vesical emptying and bacterial growth on the mechanism of bladder defense to infection	J Urol 1961, 86, 739
25	236	Leadbetter	Hypertension in unilateral renal disease	J Urol 1938, 39, 611
26	234	Marshall	The relation of the preoperative estimate to the pathologic demonstration of the extent of vesical neoplasms	J Urol 1952, 68, 714
27	234	**Berry SJ**	**The development of human benign prostatic hyperplasia with age**	**J Urol 1984, 132, 474**
28	230	Lapides J	Structure and function of the internal vesical sphincter	J Urol 1958, 80, 341
29	229	Althausen	Non-invasive papillary carcinoma of the bladder associated with carcinoma in situ	J Urol 1976, 116, 575
30	229	**Heney MM**	**Superficial bladder cancer – progression and recurrence**	**J Urol 1983, 130, 1083**

31	229	Riches EW	New growths of the kidney and ureter	Brit J Urol 1951, 23, 297
32	228	Lue TF	Physiology of erection and pharmacological management of impotence	J Urol 1987, 137, 829
33	225	Whitaker	Methods of assessing obstruction in dilated ureters	Brit J Urol 1973, 45, 15
34	223	Walsh PC	Impotence following radical prostatectomy – insight into etiology and prevention	J Urol 1982, 128, 492
35	221	Smith HW	Unilateral nephrectomy in hypertensive disease	J Urol 1956, 76, 685
36	220	Zorgniotti	Auto-injection of the corpus cavernosum with a vasoactive drug-combination for vasculogenic impotence	J Urol 1985, 133, 39
37	214	Hudson MA	Clinical use of prostate specific antigen in patients with prostate cancer	J Urol 1989, 142, 1011
38	210	Middleton	Surgery for metastatic renal cell carcinoma	J Urol 1967, 97, 973
39	210	Robertson	Risk factors in calcium stone disease	Brit J Urol 1978, 50, 449
40	210	Fowler JE	**Studies of introital colonization in women with recurrent urinary tract infections. vii. The role of bacterial adherence**	**J Urol 1977, 117, 472–476**
41	207	Decenzo JM	Antigenic deletion and prognosis of patients with stage A transitional cell bladder carcinoma	J Urol 1975, 114, 874
42	207	Lange PH	The value of serum prostate specific antigen determinations before and after radical prostatectomy	J Urol 1989, 141, 873
43	205	Paquin AJ	Ureterovesical anastomosis: the description and evaluation of a technique	J Urol 1959, 82, 573
44	201	Moore RA	The morphology of small prostatic carcinoma	J Urol 1935, 33, 224
45	**201**	**Walsh PC**	**Radical prostatectomy with preservation of sexual function – anatomical and pathological considerations**	**Prostate 1983, 4, 473**
46	201	Winter CC	A clinical study of a new function test: the radioactive Diodrast renogram	J Urol 1956, 76, 182
47	200	Brosman SA	Experience with Bacillus Calmette–Guérin in patients with superficial bladder carcinoma	J Urol 1982, 128, 27
48	**199**	**Scott FB**	**Management of erectile impotence use of implantable inflatable prosthesis**	**Urology 1973, 2, 80–82**
49	196	Herring LC	Observations on the analysis of ten thousand urinary calculi	J Urol 1962, 88, 545

#	Author	Title		Reference
50	Almgard LE	Treatment of renal adenocarcinomas by embolic occlusion of the renal circulation	193	Brit J Urol 1973, 45, 474
51	Bates P	The standardization of terminology of lower urinary tract function	192	J Urol 1979, 121, 551
52	Cantrell BB	Pathological factors that influence prognosis in stage a prostatic cancer – the influence of extent versus grade	191	J Urol 1981, 125, 516
53	Melicow MM	Histological study of vesical urothelium intervening between gross neoplasms in total cystectomy	189	J Urol 1952, 68, 261
54	Sternberg	Preliminary results of M-VAC (methotrexate, vinblastine, doxorubicin and cisplatin) for transitional cell carcinoma of the urothelium	189	J Urol 1985, 133, 403
55	DeKernion	The natural history of metastatic renal cell carcinoma: a computer analysis	187	J Urol 1978, 120, 148
56	Barzell W	Prostatic adenocarcinoma: relationship of grade and local extent to the pattern of metastases	185	J Urol 1977, 118, 278
57	Shapiro SR	Fate of 90 children with ileum conduit urinary diversion a decade later: analysis of complications, pyelography, renal function and bacteriology	184	J Urol 1975, 114, 289
58	Stamey TA	Morphometric and clinical studies on 68 consecutive radical prostatectomies	182	J Urol 1988, 139, 1235
59	Bors E	Neurological disturbances of sexual function with special reference to 529 patients with spinal cord injuries	181	Urol Surv 1960, 10, 191
60	Caine M	Adrenergic and cholinergic receptors in the human prostate, prostatic capsule and bladder neck	181	Brit J Urol 1975, 47, 193
61	Stamey TA	Prostate specific antigen in the diagnosis and treatment of adenocarcinoma of the prostate. I. untreated patients	181	J Urol 1989, 141, 1070
62	Partin A W	Prostate specific antigen in the staging of localized prostate cancer – influence of tumor differentiation, tumor volume and benign hyperplasia	179	J Urol 1990, 143, 747
63	Collins DH	Results of treatment of uretero-pelvic junction obstruction	178	Brit J Urol 1964, 36, 1
64	**McGuire EJ**	**Prognostic value of urodynamic testing in myelodysplastic patients**	**178**	**J Urol 1981, 126, 205**
65	Paulson DF	Radical surgery versus radiotherapy for adenocarcinoma of the prostate	178	J Urol 1982, 128, 502
66	Labrie F	New approach in the treatment of prostate cancer – complete instead of partial withdrawal of androgens	175	Prostate 1983, 4, 579

67	175	Whitmore	Radical cystectomy with or without prior irradiation in the treatment of bladder cancer	J Urol 1977, 118, 184
68	174	Rich AR	On the frequency of occurrence of occult carcinoma of the prostate	J Urol 1935, 33, 215
69	174	Skinner DG	Extension of renal cell carcinoma into the vena cava: the rationale for aggressive surgical management	J Urol 1972, 107, 711
70	173	Esposti	Cytologic malignancy grading of prostatic carcinoma by transrectal biopsy	Scand J Urol Nephrol 1971, 5, 199
71	173	Kelly JF	Hematoporphyrin derivative: a possible aid in the diagnosis and therapy of carcinoma of the bladder	J Urol 1976, 115, 150
72	173	McLaughlin	Prostatic carcinoma: incidence and location of unsuspected lymphatic metastases	J Urol 1976, 115, 89
73	171	Donker PJ	Analyses of the urethral pressure profile by means of electromyography and the administration of drugs	Brit J Urol 1972, 44, 180
74	171	Lutzeyer W	Prognostic parameters in superficial bladder cancer – an analysis of 315 cases	J Urol 1982, 127, 250
75	**170**	**Sternberg**	**M-VAC (methotrexate, vinblastine, doxorubicin and cisplatin) for advanced transitional cell carcinoma of the urothelium**	**J Urol 1988, 139, 461**
76	170	Whitmore	Radical total cystectomy for cancer of the bladder: 230 consecutive cases five years later	J Urol 1962, 87, 853
77	168	Boyce WH	The amount and nature of the organic matrix in urinary calculi: a review	J Urol 1956, 76, 213
78	167	Tribukait B	The significance of ploidy and proliferation in the clinical and biological evaluation of bladder tumors – a study of 100 untreated cases	Brit J Urol 1982, 54, 130
79	165	Chaussy C	Extracorporeal shock-wave lithotripsy (ESWL) for treatment of urolithiasis	Urology 1984, 23, 59
80	165	Macleod J	The male factor in fertility and infertility. II. Spermatozoon counts in 1000 men of known fertility and in 1000 cases of infertile marriage	J Urol 1951, 66, 436
81	163	Schmidt JD	Complications, results and problems of ileal conduit diversions	J Urol 1973, 109, 210
82	162	Flocks RH	Lymphatic spread from prostatic cancer	J Urol 1959, 81, 194
83	161	Lue TF	Hemodynamics of erection in the monkey	J Urol 1983, 130, 1237
84	160	Tribukait B	Flow cytometry in assessing the clinical aggressiveness of genitourinary neoplasms	World J Urol 1987, 5, 108

85	159	Lange PH	Tissue blood-group antigens and prognosis in low stage transitional cell carcinoma of the bladder	J Urol 1978, 119, 52
86	158	Bloom HJG	Treatment of T3 bladder cancer – controlled trial of pre-operative radiotherapy and radical cystectomy versus radical radiotherapy – 2nd report and review for the Clinical Trials Group, Institute of Urology	Brit J Urol 1982, 54, 136
87	158	Ercole CJ	Prostatic specific antigen and prostatic acid-phosphatase in the monitoring and staging of patients with prostatic cancer	J Urol 1987, 138, 1181
88	155	Beck AD	The effect of intra-uterine urinary obstruction upon the development of the fetal kidney	J Urol 1971, 105, 784
89	156	Greene LF	Benign papilloma or papillary carcinoma of the bladder?	J Urol 1973, 110, 205
90	154	Lingeman JE	Extracorporeal shock-wave lithotripsy – the Methodist Hospital of Indiana experience	J Urol 1986, 135, 1134
91	153	Lamm DL	Bacillus Calmette–Guérin immunotherapy for bladder cancer	J Urol 1985, 134, 40
92	153	Scardino PT	The value of serum tumor markers in the staging and prognosis of germ cell tumors of the testis	J Urol 1977, 118, 994
93	151	Bors E	Neurogenic bladder	Urol Surv 1957, 7, 177
94	151	O'Reilly PH	Diuresis renography in equivocal urinary tract obstruction	Brit J Urol 1978, 50, 76
95	150	Lamm DL	Complications of Bacillus Calmette–Guérin immunotherapy in 1,278 patients with bladder cancer	J Urol 1986, 135, 272
96	150	Wallace DM	The management of deeply infiltrating (T3) bladder carcinoma: Controlled trial of radical radiotherapy versus preoperative radiotherapy and radical cystectomy (first report)	Brit J Urol 1976, 48, 587
97	149	Bengtsson	Transitional cell tumors of the renal pelvis in analgesic abusers	Scand J Urol Nephrol 1968, 2, 145
98	149	Murphy GP	The national survey of prostate cancer in the United States by the American College of Surgeons	J Urol 1982, 127, 928
99	148	Epstein JI	Prognosis of untreated stage-A1 prostatic carcinoma – a study of 94 cases with extended follow-up	J Urol 1986, 136, 837
100	**147**	**Fernstrom I**	**Percutaneous pyelolithotomy: a new extraction technique**	**Scand J Urol Nephrol 1976, 10, 257–259**

* Citation counts provided by ISI.
† The database from which this information was taken was not able to supply all paper titles.

Table 3: Citation counts of papers appearing in *Classic Papers in Urology* combined with papers appearing in Tables 1 and 2 *†

Bold text = paper appears in *Classic Papers in Urology*

Position	Citation count	Author	Paper title	Journal, date, volume, page no.
1	1096	**Einhorn & Donohue**	**Cis diaminochloroplatinum, vinblastine, and bleomycin combination chemotherapy in disseminated testicular cancer**	**Annals of Internal Medicine 1977, 87, 293–298**
2	1037	**Huggins & Hodges**	**Studies on prostate cancer. The effect of castration, of estrogen and of androgen injection on serum phosphatases in metastatic carcinoma of the prostate.**	**Cancer Research 1941, I, 293–297**
3	870	**Stamey et al**	**Prostate specific antigen as a serum marker for adenocarcinoma of the prostate**	**New England J Medicine 1987, 317, 909–916**
4	538	Oesterling JE	Prostate specific antigen – a critical assessment of the most useful tumor marker for adenocarcinoma of the prostate	J Urol 1991, 145, 907
5	528	**Kass & Finland**	**Asymptomatic infections of the urinary tract**	**Trans Association Am Physicians 1956, 69, 56**
6	498	**Robson et al**	**The results of radical nephrectomy for renal cell carcinoma**	**J Urol 1969, 101, 297–301**
7	472	Gleason DF	Prediction of prognosis for prostatic adenocarcinoma by combined histological grading and clinical staging	J Urol 1974, 111, 58
8	465	**Mebust et al**	**Transurethral prostatectomy: immediate and post-operative complications. A co-operative study of 13 participating institutions evaluating 3,885 patients.**	**J Urol 1989, 141, 243–247**
9	415	**Bricker**	**Bladder substitution after pelvic evisceration**	**Surg Clin North Amer 1950, 30, 1511–1521**
10	404	**Politano & Leadbetter**	**An operative technique for the correction of vesicoureteral reflux**	**J Urol 1958, 79, 932–941**
11	399	Jewett HJ	Infiltrating carcinoma of the bladder. Relation of depth of penetration of the bladder wall to incidence of local extension and metastases	J Urol 1946, 55, 366
12	388	**Berry et al**	**The development of human benign prostatic hyperplasia with age**	**J Urol 1984, 132, 474–479**
13	384	Stamey TA	Prostate specific antigen in the diagnosis and treatment of adenocarcinoma of the prostate. 2. Radical prostatectomy treated patients	J Urol 1989, 141, 1076

	Author	Title	Reference
14	Herbut P	†	In, Myron Tannebaum (Editor) Urological Pathology, Lea & Febiger, Philadelphia, 1977
15	Schwartz et al	A simple estimation of glomerular filtration rate in children derived from body length and plasma creatinine	Pediatrics 1976, 58, 259–263
16	Gleason DF & the VACURG	Histologic grading and clinical staging of prostate carcinoma	In, Myron Tannebaum (Editor) Urological Pathology, Lea & Febiger, Philadelphia, 1977, 171–197
17	Oesterling JE	Prostate specific antigen in the pre-operative and post-operative evaluation of localized prostatic cancer treated with radical prostatectomy	J Urol 1988, 139, 766
18	Roos et al	Mortality and re-operation after open and transurethral resection of the prostate for benign prostatic hyperplasia	New England Journal of Medicine 1989, 320, 1120–1124
19	Crawford et al	A controlled trial of leuprolide with and without flutamide in prostatic carcinoma	New England J Medicine 1989, 321, 419–424
20	Ormond JK	Bilateral ureteral obstruction due to envelopment and compression by an inflammatory retroperitoneal process	J Urol 1948, 59, 1072
21	Cooner WH	Prostate cancer detection in a clinical urological practice by ultrasonography, digital rectal examination and prostate specific antigen	J Urol 1990, 143, 1146
22	Virag	Intracavernous injection of papaverine for erectile failure	The Lancet, 1982, Oct. 23, 938.
23	Johansson et al	High 10 year survival rate in patients with early untreated prostate cancer	JAMA 1992, 267, 2191–2196
24	Berger J	Les depots intercapillaires d'IgA–IgG	J Urologie 1968, 74, 694
25	Brown M	The urethral pressure profile	Brit J Urol 1969, 41, 211
26	Drach GW	Report of the United States cooperative study of extracorporeal shock-wave lithotripsy	J Urol 1986, 135, 1127
27	Lange PH	The value of serum prostate specific antigen determinations before and after radical prostatectomy	J Urol 1989, 141, 873
28	Morales A et al	Intracavitary Bacillus Calmette–Guérin in the treatment of superficial bladder tumours	J Urol 1976, 116, 180–183

No	Author	Title	Reference	Page
29	Barry et al	The American Urological Association symptom index for benign prostatic hyperplasia	J Urol 1992, 148, 1549–1557	315
30	Catalona et al	Detection of organ confined prostate cancer is increased through prostate specific antigen based screening	JAMA 1993, 270, 948–954	315
31	Hudson MA	Clinical use of prostate specific antigen in patients with prostate cancer	J Urol 1989, 142, 1011	315
32	Chaussy et al	Extracorporeal shock wave lithotrypsy	The Lancet 1980, 2, 1265–1268	314
33	Chaussy C	1st clinical experience with extracorporeally induced destruction of kidney stones by shock-waves	J Urol 1982, 127, 417	314
34	Stamm et al	Diagnosis of coliform infection in acutely dysuric women	New England J Urol 1982, 307, 463–468	313
35	Franzen S	Cytological diagnosis of prostatic tumours by transrectal aspiration biopsy: a preliminary report	Brit J Urol 1960, 32, 193	308
36	Lue TF	Physiology of erection and pharmacological management of impotence	J Urol 1987, 137, 829	307
37	Heney et al	Superficial bladder cancer: progression and recurrence	J Urol 1983, 130, 1083–1086	303
38	Meares & Stamey	Bacteriologic localization patterns in bacterial prostatitis and urethritis	Investigative Urology 1968, 5, 492–518	302
39	Walsh PC	Impotence following radical prostatectomy – insight into etiology and prevention	J Urol 1982, 128 492	293
40	Kock et al	Urinary diversion via a continent ileal reservoir: clinical results in twelve patients	J Urol 1982, 128, 469–475	289
41	Stamey TA	Prostate specific antigen in the diagnosis and treatment of adenocarcinoma of the prostate. 2. Radical prostatectomy treated patients	J Urol 1989, 141, 1076	286
42	Catalona WJ	Comparison of digital rectal examination and serum prostate-specific antigen in the early detection of prostate cancer – results of a multicenter clinical trial of 6,630 men	J Urol 1994, 151, 1283	284
43	Jewett HJ	The present status of radical prostatectomy for stages A and B prostatic cancer	Urol Clin N Am 1975, 2, 105	284
44	Partin W	Prostate specific antigen in the staging of localized prostate cancer – influence of tumor differentiation, tumor volume and benign hyperplasia	J Urol 1990, 143, 747	283

#		Author	Title	Reference
45	282	Prien EL	Studies in urolithiasis: I. The composition of urinary calculi	J Urol 1947, 57, 949
46	277	Partin AW	The use of prostate-specific antigen, clinical stage and Gleason score to predict pathological stage in men with localized prostate cancer	J Urol 1993, 150, 110
47	267	Brawer MK	Screening for prostatic carcinoma with prostate specific antigen	J Urol 1992, 147, 841
48	262	Lapides J et al	Clean intermittent self-catheterization in the treatment of urinary tract disease	J Urol 1972, 107, 458–461
49	262	Zorgniotti AW	Auto-injection of the corpus cavernosum with a vasoactive drug-combination for vasculogenic impotence	J Urol 1985, 133, 39
50	261	D'Angio et al	The treatment of Wilms tumor – results of the National Wilms Tumor Study	Cancer 1976, 38, 633–646
51	258	Christensson A	Serum prostate-specific antigen complexed to alpha-1–antichymotrypsin as an indicator of prostate cancer	J Urol 1993, 150, 100
52	255	Mostofi FK	Potentialities of bladder urothelium	J Urol 1954, 71, 705
53	253	Benson MC	The use of prostate specific antigen density to enhance the predictive value of intermediate levels of serum prostate specific antigen	J Urol 1992, 147, 817
54	246	McGuire et al	Prognostic value of urodynamic testing in myelodysplastic patients	J Urol 1981, 126, 205–209
55	246	Walsh et al	Radical prostatectomy with preservation of sexual function: anatomical and pathological considerations	The Prostate 1983, 4, 473–485
56	237	Ignarro et al	Nitric oxide and cyclic GMP formation upon electrical field stimulation cause relaxation of corpus cavernosum smooth muscle	Biochemical and Biophysical Research Communications 1990, 170, 843–850
57	237	Stamey TA	Morphometric and clinical studies on 68 consecutive radical prostatectomies	J Urol 1988, 139, 1235
58	236	Cox CE	Experiments with induced bacteriuria, vesical emptying and bacterial growth on the mechanism of bladder defense in infection	J Urol 1961, 86, 739
59	236	Leadbetter	Hypertension in unilateral renal disease	J Urol 1938, 39, 611
60	234	Burch	Urethrovaginal fixation to Cooper's ligament for correction of stress incontinence, cystocele, and prolapse	American Journal of Obstetrics & Gynecology 1961, 81, 281–290
61	234	Marshall	The relation of the preoperative estimate to the pathologic demonstration of the extent of vesical neoplasms	J Urol 1952, 68, 714

62	Lapides J	Structure and function of the internal vesical sphincter	J Urol 1958, 80, 341
63	Althausen	Non-invasive papillary carcinoma of the bladder associated with carcinoma in situ	J Urol 1976, 116, 575
64	Riches EW	New growths of kidney and ureter	Brit J Urol 1951, 23, 297
65	Benson MC	Prostate specific antigen density – a means of distinguishing benign prostatic hypertrophy and prostate cancer	J Urol 1992, 147, 815
66	Whitaker	Methods of assessing obstruction in dilated ureters	Brit J Urol 1973, 45, 15
67	Sternberg CN	Preliminary results of M-VAC (methotrexate, vinblastine, doxorubicin and cisplatin) for transitional cell carcinoma of the urothelium	J Urol 1985, 133, 403
68	**Mitrofanoff**	**Cystostomie continente trans-appendiculaire dans le traitment des vessies neurologiques**	**Chir Pediatr (Paris) 1980, 21, 297–305**
69	Partin AW	Serum PSA after anatomic radical prostatectomy – the Johns Hopkins experience after 10 years	Urol Clin N Am 1993, 20, 713
70	Walsh PC	Impotence following radical prostatectomy – insight into etiology and prevention	J Urol 1982, 128, 492
71	Smith HW	Unilateral nephrectomy in hypertensive disease	J Urol 1956, 76, 685
72	**Sternberg et al**	**M-VAC (Methotrexate, vinblastine, doxorubicin and cisplatin) for advanced transitional cell carcinoma of the urothelium**	**J Urol 1988, 139, 461–469**
73	Brosman SA	Experience with Bacillus Calmette–Guérin in patients with superficial bladder carcinoma	J Urol 1982, 128, 27
74	Zorgniotti	Auto-injection of the corpus cavernosum with a vasoactive drug-combination for vasculogenic impotence	J Urol 1985, 133, 39
75	**Fowler & Stamey**	**Studies of introital colonization in women with recurrent urinary tract infections. vii. The role of bacterial adherence**	**J Urol 1977, 117, 472–476**
76	Middleton	Surgery for metastatic renal cell carcinoma	J Urol 1967, 97, 973
77	Robertson	Risk factors in calcium stone disease of the urinary tract	Brit J Urol 1978, 50, 449
78	Cantrell BB	Pathological factors that influence prognosis in stage a prostatic cancer – the influence of extent versus grade	J Urol 1981, 125, 516
79	Paulson DF	Radical surgery versus radiotherapy for adenocarcinoma of the prostate	J Urol 1982, 128, 502

#	Page	Author	Title	Citation
80	207	Decenzo JM	Antigenic deletion and prognosis of patients with stage A transitional cell bladder carcinoma	J Urol 1975, 114, 874
81	207	Lange PH	The value of serum prostate specific antigen determinations before and after radical prostatectomy	J Urol 1989, 141, 873
82	207	Stamey TA	Prostate specific antigen in the diagnosis and treatment of adenocarcinoma of the prostate. I. untreated patients	J Urol 1989, 141, 1070
83	206	**McNeal**	**Origin and development of carcinoma of the prostate**	**Cancer 1969, 23, 24–33**
84	205	Paquin AJ	Ureterovesical anastomosis: the description and evaluation of a technique	J Urol 1959, 82, 573
85	204	**Whitmore Jr**	**The natural history of prostate cancer**	**Cancer 1973, 32, 1104–1112**
86	202	**Slater**	**Rubber anaphylaxis**	**New England J Medicine 1989, 320, 1126–1130**
87	201	Moore RA	The morphology of small prostatic carcinoma	J Urol 1935, 33, 224
88	201	**Walsh PC**	**Radical prostatectomy with preservation of sexual function – anatomical and pathological considerations**	**Prostate 1983, 4, 473**
89	201	Winter CC	A clinical study of a new renal function test: the radioactive diodrast renogram	J Urol 1956, 76, 182
90	199	**Scott FB**	**Management of erectile impotence use of implantable inflatable prosthesis**	**Urology 1973, 2, 80–82**
91	199	Hodge KK	Random systematic versus directed ultrasound guided trans-rectal core biopsies of the prostate	J Urol 1989, 142, 71
92	198	Ercole CJ	Prostate specific antigen and prostatic acid-phosphatase in the monitoring and staging of patients with prostatic cancer	J Urol 1987, 138, 1181
93	197	Schreiber MJ	The natural history of atherosclerotic and fibrous renal artery disease	Urol Clin N 1984, 11, 383
94	196	Herring LC	Observations on the analysis of ten thousand urinary calculi	J Urol 1962, 88, 545
95	196	Labrie F	New approach in the treatment of prostate cancer – complete instead of partial withdrawal of androgens	Prostate 1983, 4, 579
96	194	**Enhörning G**	**Simultaneous recording of intravesical and intraurethral pressure**	**Act Chir Scand 1961, 276, 1–68**
97	193	Almgard LE	Treatment of renal adenocarcinomas by embolic occlusion of the renal circulation	Brit J Urol 1973, 45, 474

98	Bates P	19	The standardization of terminology of lower urinary tract function	J Urol 1979, 121, 551
99	Lutzeyer W	191	Prognostic parameters in superficial bladder cancer – and analysis of 315 cases	J Urol 1982, 127, 250
100	Melicow MM	189	Histological study of vesical urothelium intervening between gross neoplasms in total cystectomy	J Urol 1952, 68, 261

* Citation counts provided by ISI.
† We were unable to find citation counts for the following papers:

- Hendren: Reconstruction of previously diverted urinary tracts in children. J Ped Surg 1973; 8: 135–150
- Karakan: A simple and inexpensive transducer for quantitative measurements of penile erection during sleep. Behav Res Meth & Instru: 1969; 1 (7): 251–252
- Simms: On the treatment of vesico-vaginal fistula. American Journal of the Medical Sciences 1852; 23: 59

No inference should be drawn from their non-appearance in this table.

INDEX

'Classic Papers' by chapter

7

8

9

10

11

12

13

14

15

'Classic Papers' by title